D0207606

Also by Donna Marie Williams

BLACK-EYED PEAS FOR THE SOUL

SISTER FEELGOOD

THE WAY OF THE BOOTSTRAPPER (*with Floyd H. Flake*)

Sensual Celibacy

THE SEXY WOMAN'S GUIDE TO
USING ABSTINENCE FOR RECHARGING
YOUR SPIRIT ✦ DISCOVERING YOUR
PASSION ✦ ACHIEVING GREATER INTIMACY
IN YOUR NEXT RELATIONSHIP

Donna Marie Williams

A Fireside Book
PUBLISHED BY SIMON & SCHUSTER

To Denise, Gino, Janice,

Karen, Laura, and Lynne

FIRESIDE
Rockefeller Center
1230 Avenue of the Americas
New York, NY 10020

Copyright © 1999 by Donna Marie Williams
All rights reserved, including the right of reproduction in whole or in part in any form.

FIRESIDE and colophon are registered trademarks of Simon & Schuster Inc.

Designed by Gretchen Achilles

Manufactured in the United States of America

10 9 8 7 6 5 4 3 2 1

Library of Congress Cataloging-in-Publication Data

Williams, Donna Marie.
Sensual celibacy : the sexy woman's guide to using abstinence for recharging your spirit, discovering your passion, achieving greater intimacy in your next relationship / Donna Marie Williams.
p. cm.
"A Fireside book."
1. Sexual ethics for women. 2. Women—Sexual behavior. 3. Chastity. 4. Man-woman relationships. I. Title.
HQ46.W55 1999
306.7'082—dc21   98-49968   CIP
ISBN 0-684-83351-4

ACKNOWLEDGMENTS

Sensual Celibacy wasn't the easiest book to write. I had to put so much of my business out on the street, and for a private person, that was painful at times. Thank goodness for my wonderful family and friends, who supported me every step of the way: Laura Williams, Janice Williams, George and Hyacinth Williams, Gino McLachlan, Lynne and Jeffrey Speller, Barry Speller, Charlie and Denise Wimberly, Larry Whitman, and Alfred "Coach" Powell.

A special thanks to the many women—single and married, religious and secular—who shared with me their stories and insights about celibacy, love, sex, men, and relationships. You taught me much.

My editors, Dawn Daniels and Becky Cabaza, are strong women of courage who took a chance on a subject that others had rejected.

And to my children, Michael and Ayanna, I pray that this book does not cause you undue embarrassment. I pray that one day you'll understand why I had to share my story with other women. I love you with all my heart and soul.

All praises to God, Jesus, and the Holy Spirit, the divine energy that flows through and connects us all.

CONTENTS

Although I do not participate in any organized form of religion, I am a Christian. Please do not feel offended if, from time to time, I use Christian terminology. I reserve the right to speak from my belief system. I honor all positive religions and belief systems and encourage you to substitute your own sacred words where applicable.

Introduction

Sex has been domesticated, stripped of the promised mystery, added to the category of the merely expected. It's just what is done, mundane as hockey. It's celibacy these days that would raise eyebrows.

—"True Trash," in *Wilderness Tips*
by Margaret Atwood

♦ ♦ ♦

I saw my first shooting star when I was about thirty-five years old. I was attending a publishing institute at Stanford University, and it was the final evening event of the most exciting two weeks of my writing and publishing career. Getting to know writers, editors, and other professionals from around the world confirmed for me that I was on the right path. I felt motivated and was anxious to get back to Chicago to put pen to paper and get busy. So on that momentous last night in California when I just happened to look up into the heavens and see that diamond light arc against the velvet black sky, I felt that the windows of heaven had opened to a new and exciting chapter in my life. No one else saw it, so I knew that the star shot across the sky for me and me alone.

Frantically I tried to remember the purpose of shooting stars from myths and legends. A wish! I had to make a wish! The universe was giving me a present, and I felt the pressure to wish wisely. I couldn't fritter away a wish on something stupid. Who knew when, or if, I'd ever get to see another one?

All the magic and wonder of the universe at my disposal and what did I wish for? A million dollars? A big house? Fame? A personal trainer? No.

I begged the universe for a husband.

The Hidden Blessing

Lord knows I could never be a nun. Although I love the idea of daily communion with the Divine, I absolutely abhor the idea of a lifelong commitment to celibacy. No men? At all? *Ever?* Just the thought makes me want to reach for the Prozac. An entire life without sex would be like a menstrual cycle without brownies and ice cream.

I am an earthy one-man woman. When I'm in a relationship with a man who excites me mentally, emotionally, spiritually, and physically, I don't care how busy I am, I'll make time for him. I love my women friends, but only Man can jump-start my heart and body in that special way that makes the sun shine, the moon glow, and the birds sing their sweet songs. I love the harshness of Man's voice, the rough feel of his day-old beard growth on my cheek when he kisses me. I love his tender (or crushing) embrace.

As much trouble as men have caused me in the past, I still crave them. Men are so habit-forming, so delicious. That's why, in times past, when I experienced the breakup of a love relationship, the idea of becoming celibate would leave me feeling anxious and depressed, sometimes for months. There were times when I didn't know what I'd miss more—the man or his you-know-what. Just like a character in a movie who's been hit with some devastating news, I'd look to heaven and scream, *"No!"* the word echoing throughout the city while the world, along with my hopes and dreams, spirals violently away into the cosmos. *"Not again!"* In times past, the onset of celibacy was, for me, like the flu; I'd feel the chills and the scratchy throat coming on, but not even a hefty dose of Nyquil (or feverish begging to please please stay) would prevent the listlessness and sadness. It was all I could do to hide under the covers and ride it through as best I could.

In times past, I haven't gone easily into that good night of celibacy. I've raged, raged against the dying light of wild and lovely sex and the energy of Man. Forget that the relationships themselves were often unfulfilling; at least I was having sex. At least I could feel romantic and in love. At least, in the harsh, judgmental eyes of society, I was a desirable woman, because I was with a man and we were having sex.

Prior to the 1960s, women were expected to stay virgins or practice celibacy if they were not married. Today, women are laughed at or pitied for choosing abstinence if they are not married, or at least in a committed, monogamous relationship. The present-day American obsession with sex has, I hate to admit, affected my beliefs about my womanhood, femininity, and celibacy. In times past, the presence of sex in my life meant that I was a full-fledged, card-carrying woman who could hold her head up high in society and among other women. The absence of sex meant no passion, no romance, no love in my life, and bowls of my father's chili to keep me company on lonely Saturday nights. Celibacy was a void—empty and utterly useless.

During periods of celibacy, which I have experienced frequently and for long durations throughout my forty years, I would nourish the idea that "spinsterhood" was my destiny with tears and negative self-talk. In my soul grew a weight as heavy and destructive as a tumor. It sabotaged one relationship that had much potential and kept me from recognizing and choosing men who were good for me. I ended up having two children by different men and under traumatic circumstances.

Celibacy was like a prison, and all I could think of was escape. "Get back into a relationship and quick" was my mantra. My manhunt was tainted by desperation and humiliation and would usually lead to involvements with men who were great in bed but bad to the bone. Despite all the obvious signs, I would get involved just to take the edge off the loneliness. Since my moral code and psychological makeup dictate that I *be* in love before I *make* love, I would usually use my fertile imagination to convince myself that I had met my prince.

In my love relationships, however, Truth takes no prisoners. Truth always wins out and destroys the fantasies, the lies. I might not have always known it, but breakups have been a blessing. While I may have been willing to settle for men who were no good for me, my God wanted the best for me. Breakups that I thought were divine punishment for having sex outside of marriage in the first place (that old Christian programming dies hard) were really opportunities to heal negative subconscious psychological patterns, destructive behaviors, and my dysfunctional approach to relationships. Breakups, and ultimately celibacy, gained me a greater understanding of my life purpose and an unconditional love for myself.

Throughout my adult life I have returned to celibacy time and again. In fact, I have been celibate more than I have been sexually active—which isn't easy for a romantic, passionate woman like me. When a woman finds herself alone in this society, too often her feminine soul suffers in shame, loneliness, and despair. When we vent with our sister-friends, we lament about how that man done did us wrong, but deep down, what we're really feeling is a profound lack of self-worth. We, in our solitude, feel totally alone in the world. We may imagine the whole world as a married couple having sex. During some of my worst moments, I felt as if my naked ring finger revealed all my fears and insecurities to the world. I felt I was on public display. "Look at her," I imagined people were saying, "no ring! She can't even keep a man. She's an incompetent woman. She's not pretty. She's not desirable." And the worst blow of all, *"She's not lovable."*

Late bloomer that I am, I was about thirty-four years old and just had Baby #2 outside of marriage when I became conscious of that last fear. I was forced to rethink all my beliefs and values. I discovered that I had made the classic mistake so many women, young and old, make: I equated sex with love, so whenever I wasn't in a relationship, I didn't feel lovable. Even though I knew I was a good woman with a lot of heart, I doubted my worth. The problem was that my womanhood and femininity were firmly entrenched within the context of relationships with men. I had no identity or sense of worth outside my male-female relationships. Looking back, the story of my life makes sense. I never could have developed identity and self-worth within a relationship. I needed the time alone. Although I perceived celibacy as sexual famine and karmic punishment, the times alone were gold mines of opportunities to discover the real me.

I rebelled, of course, and often. Sometimes daily. I prayed, I begged, I bargained with my God to please give me a husband. I was so dependent on Man to define me that having to rely on myself was scary. At the time I didn't realize that my prayers were being answered. I couldn't see beyond the emptiness of my life and the dark, lonely void. I felt as if no man would ever love me again. Sometimes I didn't even care if *I* loved me or not.

Motherhood proved to be the blessing that set me firmly on the path of my sensual, self loving approach to celibacy. Although I did not set out to get pregnant with either of my children, I take my maternal responsibilities seriously. Whether my son and daughter were planned or not, whether they have the benefit of one full-time father or not, at the very least they deserve a good, devoted mother. As long as I'm not in a bad, emotionally draining relationship, I can be that for them.

Roller-coaster emotional entanglements negatively affect my ability to be a good mother. They leave me feeling depressed, disoriented, irritable, and tense, which, of course, taints my interaction with my children. My children are so sensitive, they often internalize my moods, which only adds to my guilt. It's not fair to my children or to me to constantly live life in a state of anxiety. We need peace. *I* need peace.

Being a new mother taught me this: The types of relationships I had settled for in the past would not serve me in my role as mother. That was a start. I wanted to be a positive role model for my children. I couldn't just have sex, hoping that the man might, maybe one day, want to possibly marry me, hopefully. I wanted my children to either see me alone, sovereign, and reasonably happy, or in a healthy, committed, loving, monogamous relationship that had marriage as a goal. I was no longer interested in trying out a guy to see if he worked. I have never, and will never, allow a parade of men into my children's lives. That would perpetuate the madness into the next generation.

We should be very selective about the men our children get to meet. Children form deep attachments to people, and when your relationship doesn't work out and the man leaves and never comes back, they experience abandonment and rejection just like you do. I've gone through enough of that, and I don't want my children to experience it unnecessarily.

And then there's my own sanity to consider. Putting my children aside for a moment, having sex with men who talk commitment but do not behave in a committed fashion (marriage) is dangerous. AIDS and STDs notwithstanding, the constant breakups take a toll on the heart. I don't have a study to back me up, but I believe depression resulting from relationship fallout is the number one health problem in this country.

Yet we keep doing the same things over and over. Our vaginas hold much power, so many of us use sex to attempt to control a man. That scheme may work temporarily, but sexual manipulation can only go so far in holding a man. In fact, the sex that we whip on a man can backfire in ways that are most unpleasant.

The spiritual mechanics of sex is a powerful process that should be taught along with the physical mechanics to every girl and boy. The womb of a woman is like a bowl; its design allows a woman to not only receive a man's sperm, but his energy, his essence into her bowl.

A man projects outward, so it takes a lot more than your good sex to keep him interested. He must receive your essence in other ways. The self-help literature does women a disservice by focusing so much on sexual technique to snare a man. According to the men I've talked to, bedroom gymnastics alone will not keep a man interested. Self-confidence, independence, good humor, and a good heart are what will keep a man's attention in the long-term.

Try this experiment: Close your eyes and focus on your pelvic area. Now do a Kegel (squeeze your vaginal muscles as if holding back urine) as deeply as you can. Hold a few seconds. If you're like me, a bolt of lightning energy will shoot straight from your womb up to your heart. When a man's penis is inside of you and you're Kegeling like crazy, simultaneously your heart is being electrically massaged and stimulated, and it's ecstasy. I don't know if that womb-heart electric connection is due to conditioning or biology, but I've learned the hard way that it's Heartbreak Hotel to mess around with it.

If I were made of stone, casual sex wouldn't be such a problem. I'm not made of stone, and you probably aren't either. When I'm turned on and my heart gets that jolt, it feels like *love*. A mere memory of an erotic experience can jolt my heart into waves of ecstasy. This feeling confused me in the past. I thought the good sex feeling *was* love. I'm one of those women (and I know I'm not alone) who has a hard time distinguishing between good sex and love. They both feel the same to me. When I first learned this about myself, I decided to become like men and learn to have sex for sex's sake. Thank goodness that foolishness was short-lived and did not lead to any sexual involvements. I have learned to accept and love my ability to receive male energy. I honor it and protect it. I now know that it's important for me to keep my queenly jewels under a lock and key of my own design until Mr. Right is doing more than just talking a good game. He's got to be willing to put in some celibacy time with me. Then he'd better get himself to the church on time because we'll have a lot of catching up to do!

*Y*OU MUSTN'T FORCE SEX TO DO THE WORK OF LOVE OR LOVE TO DO THE WORK OF SEX.
—MARY MCCARTHY

Our bowl design—our feminine ability to receive and embrace, both physically and spiritually—causes us to retain a man's energy for a long time. I have a long memory for men with whom I've been sexually involved. I still have dreams about men I broke up with years ago. I don't know if this is true for men, but I believe it is true for many of us women. Unless a woman makes the conscious decision to emotionally and psychologically heal from a broken affair, the man's lingering energy will continue to cause painful memories, which, on a downward spiral, can lead to destructive behaviors and low self-worth. I have gone through the hard healing work, and although I'll always remember incidents I wish I could forget, I've come a long way. There is absolutely no way I want to start at square one again. Thank goodness for celibacy. The horniness (to be quite blunt) I experience from time to time is a small price to pay for sanity, contentment, and peace of mind. I can handle the occasional bouts of loneliness knowing that the sun will rise and the morning will come. Until then, there's so much living to do! There's not enough time in the day to get it all done.

So I've been forced to become much more selective about men. After the birth of my daughter, my second (and last) child born outside of marriage, I knew I'd have to make some big changes in my life. My daughter's father and I tried to make it work during the first few months of her life, but the relationship was doomed from the start. Inevitably, we broke up. I just couldn't keep going on like this, making babies with (1) men I was not married to and (2) men who did not love me.

The birth of my first child left me feeling devastated and terrified. The birth of my second child woke me up. I began to realize that my approach to relationships was completely dysfunctional. It took one more failed relationship (after the one with my daughter's father) to convince me that I needed to take a break not only from sex, but from men in general. I couldn't just *be* with a man because he made me feel good, hoping against hope that love and marriage would come later. I had to develop some long-term goals and objectives apart from my desire for a mate. I would have to become a whole person, despite our society's belief that a woman is nothing without a man. I would have to get a life.

I would also have to raise my expectations of men. This was a new and frightening exercise. If men were scarce before I began to insist on character, sterling treatment, and commitment, my chances would plunge to zero if I tried to expect more from them. I had always experienced long "dry" spells between relationships, but after the birth of my children, they became longer and drier. Would I ever find love and happiness?

Wrong question. I learned to ask a better one: How do I turn the famine times into feast times? Deep down, I knew my focus had to change from men to my own healing. The exciting journey of self-discovery was what life was all about. I decided to be honest with myself about what I wanted and needed in a man, then I surrendered my search and let the helpful forces in the Universe take care of the rest. In the meantime, I had work to do. I had to switch on my internal light to find the Me I had lost in the years of bad relationships and rough periods of celibacy. I had to find the treasure that was hidden in this wilderness called celibacy, lest I go crazy. Hence, the Sensual Celibacy Program.

When my first unconscious forays into celibacy began, I was twenty-four years old, scared, newly divorced, and desperately unhappy. Apart from church teachings and Xaviera Hollander's racy books, I had little to guide me in the arena of women's sexuality. I began to rely on myself to answer questions such as: What is celibacy? What is sexuality? What is womanhood and femininity? What is passion? What is sin?

Ten years later, during my first conscious, tentative steps in this uncharted territory, I still had no clue—but at least I was awake and willing to do the hard heart work. I prayed and felt my way through the process. There was no map. There were no hip, modern, feminine, sexy role models. I don't participate in any organized religion, so there was no support group of women practicing celibacy. I could always depend on the love of my sisters and best friend, and they talked me through many a lonely, sleepless night, but as for sharing experiences with other single women, I was on my own.

I had been practicing the self-loving, productive style of celibacy for a couple of years when the term "sensual celibacy" hit me like a bolt of lightning. This is what I had been doing all along! I had been so blessed by this particular style of celibacy that I just knew I had to share it with single women who were struggling with the same issues I had been.

Why not "sensual abstinence"? According to most definitions, the word "abstinence" is a catchall for the act of self-denial. You can abstain from anything—eating red meat, drinking alcohol, and having sex. "Celibacy," on the other hand, specifically refers to abstention from sexual intercourse. The phrase "sensual celibacy" means a sexual abstention that is (1) empowering, (2) nonjudgmental, (3) healing, (4) loving, and (5) fun. The Sensual Celibacy Program is a 10-step guide that offers

skill-building exercises, self-esteem boosting affirmations, guided imagery, meditations, and self-assessments to help women make the most
out of their vacations from sex.

Celibacy is distinguished from virginity in that celibates have sam-
pled the delights of the apple. We know what we are missing; virgins do
not (more or less). In bygone eras, the term "virgin" used to refer to an
individual who was pure and innocent in spirit, but today that concept
has been narrowed to refer to an individual who has not had sexual intercourse. I like the former definition. It is more expansive, allowing for
more possibilities for self-love, self-discovery, and personal growth. In
response to high teen pregnancy rates and sexually transmitted diseases
among young people, the virginity movement appears to be gaining acceptance as a "hip" lifestyle choice. (More on the virginity movement in
chapter 11.)

In addition to abstaining from sexual intercourse, this book adds
the dimensions of *decision* and *sensuality* to today's enlightened approach
to celibacy. Realistically, I know that women will continue to have sex
without the benefit of marriage, so I add this caveat: *Celibacy is about
making the decision to abstain from sexual intercourse when there is no
healthy, loving, monogamous, committed relationship
present in your life.* Monogamy and commitment are
our base-level criteria for entering into the sexual
phase of a relationship; otherwise, it will amount to
nothing more than a casual affair. We need to get
away from casual affairs because they do not serve
the goals of women who desire marriage or a committed, monogamous
relationship. Nor do they serve the holy grail of holistic health—mind,
body, emotions, and spirit. Ultimately, I believe that in the new millennium we will see increasing numbers of women (and men) choosing
premarital celibacy as a way of reclaiming and healing their bodies,
minds, and souls.

> *L*OSING MY VIR-
> GINITY WAS A CAREER
> MOVE.
> —MADONNA

The dimension of sensuality makes this decision a pleasure, as all of
the physical and spiritual senses are celebrated rather than suppressed.
How long does a woman have to abstain from sex before she can say she
is officially practicing celibacy? Shere Hite says six months, and we will
also use that time frame as a guide.

Give Yourself a Gift

Our popular ideas and feelings about celibacy were bequeathed to us from a harsh, judgmental, intolerant era. Celibacy was a grit-your-teeth, humorless experience. The poster child for celibacy was a pale woman who wore spectacles, her hair was pulled back in a respectable bun, and her gray dress was high-necked and long-sleeved. In our age when sex is more or less a given in relationships, this image of celibacy as grim, prudish, determined, and humorless still shapes our ideas about the practice. It's just not very enticing. Sensual celibacy obliterates all those old, destructive ideas and gives us a new, more empowering way to think about celibacy.

The Sensual Celibacy Program is my gift to you. I know what women go through. I know how confused we are about love, sex, and relationships. The Program makes celibacy not only a bearable experience, but a healing, productive, and even joyous one. You'll learn that you do not have to sacrifice feelings of romance and passion just because there is no man in your life. You'll learn how to feel about yourself the way you might feel about a love interest, which means you won't have to give up the good feelings at all. You can love and romance yourself. Imagine, loving yourself as intensely as any man you've ever loved! That's hot!

My entire life and personal philosophy have changed because of my practice of celibacy. I now take myself out on dates, and I treat myself to sensual delights such as good, positive music, delicious foods, stimulating books and cultural events, and good friends. I hug and touch people more, which helps satisfy my skin's hunger and my need to connect with others. As much as possible I infuse sensuality into every aspect of my life, from the clothes I wear and the sheets I sleep in to the pictures I hang on my walls. Even my prayers are romantic and passionate. Day by day, I am learning to experience life through all my senses. Amazingly, celibacy becomes less the focal point of my existence. Life is the point.

The Program has taught me skills to strengthen my practice of celibacy, i.e., my ability to resist temptation and withstand pressure before I am fully ready to have sex. I have learned that a goal-oriented approach gives my periods of celibacy focus and purpose.

Idleness, the enemy of any celibacy practice, has no place in the Program. Idleness is different from stillness. Idleness is doing nothing; stillness is being centered and listening to your inner spirit. The Program balances activity and stillness. My days are filled with meaningful activities—not busywork—that have their source in what I currently understand is my life purpose. Many women, upon finding themselves celibate, will fill up their days with a flurry of activity. This busywork only temporarily lets them forget about their problems. Eventually, however, they will have to face the music. How to tell if you've been engaged in busywork or meaningful activity? If you can spend an entire day alone in the stillness, if you can spend quality, quiet time alone with yourself without feeling panicky, then you know the Program is working.

One of the biggest benefits of the Program is that by taking time for yourself, by honestly looking at your true desires about vocation, marriage, etc., you'll begin to get some inkling of your life purpose. Inside many a computer programmer or secretary or doctor beats the heart of an artist or educator. Some of us are supposed to be wives and mothers, but because of the stigma attached to that honorable profession, the calling has been denied. How can you know if you never take the time to find out?

Before I started the Program, I was bored all the time. Since I made my first conscious decision to practice celibacy, which was about two years after the birth of my second child, I can honestly say that I have not experienced one dull moment. Life has been full, rich, and meaningful because my activities are now grounded in life-mission work.

Another miracle has happened too: While I still need Man (after all, I am Woman), I need him in a different way. I need friendship, communication, and empathy from him. I will always crave intimacy with a man, but now I know I don't have to have sex to experience the feelings (although sex would be nice). I can be in a business meeting and satisfy my need for Man just by being in his company. This has freed me to experience men as human beings, not as penis machines. I have real friendships with men now, something I never had before.

As most women know, sex is plentiful and easily available, if that's all that's desired. Since most of us want more than just an uncommitted, unfulfilling toss in the hay, today's celibate women and men are consciously deciding to abstain from sex for self-determined periods of time. Making the decision to forgo sex for a while is different from simply not having sex while waiting for the next lay. According to this definition, it might have been a year since you last had sex, but you are not celibate if you are in constant, hot pursuit of your next conquest. Decision makes the mechanics of celibacy (no intercourse) a much more empowering, disciplined, emotionally satisfying experience. If you've just become single, if you anticipate becoming single soon, or even if you've been resisting your celibate state for quite a while, take that first step and make the decision to become celibate. This step will be the first of many in your journey toward self-discovery. If you are single and alone, deciding to become celibate is one of the greatest acts of self-love you will ever make. A word of warning though: Don't be surprised if your entire life turns upside down!

Women need guidance on how to channel earthiness into areas other than sex. We don't need condemnation for having a vital and powerful life force. We don't need teachings that show us how to beat the flesh into submission. Throughout the Program, we will explore ways to reunite natural earthiness to spirituality, love for the environment, passion for work, health and fitness efforts, and more.

Quiet as it's kept, the church mothers and fathers talk a lot about the "sin" of "fornication," but they don't teach their single members how to matriculate through celibacy. The reality of a celibate's life is that you get horny. You get lonely. What do you do with the feelings? When I was in the church, married men and women would teach us single folks to read our Bible and just say no to sex, no to masturbation. We were taught to have faith that God would provide our mates. In fact, there was an obsessive focus on "believing in God for your mate." I recently heard of a church in which teenagers are being taught to pray to God for their mates! I love my faith, but some church teachings hurt more than help. How about teaching teens to pray to God for guidance on their life purpose and having a fulfilling, satisfying life—with or without a mate? Even though most of us want to be in a relationship, when we obsess about it, we lose perspective. The Sensual Celibacy Program puts us on the right track. When friendship, love, romance, marriage, and sex occur (hopefully in that order), you'll enter that special relationship as a whole person, not as someone needing another for completion.

Fornication, chastity, promiscuity, and *purity* are words that smack of intolerance and judgment. The old view says that celibates are chaste and pure. Sex outside of marriage is not just sex, it's fornication and promiscuity. Some even go so far as to say that single women who are having sex are whores. Yet to say that sex outside of marriage is impure implies that sex within marriage is automatically holy, and that's not necessarily the case. Just ask any woman who is repeatedly beaten and raped by her husband, or a man whose sexual relations with his wife leave him feeling emasculated. On the other hand, singles who engage in unprotected sex with multiple partners are not only putting their own lives and the lives of others in danger, they are creating layer upon layer of spiritual, emotional, and psychological problems that are seething just beneath the surface, waiting to erupt. They may claim that they love sex, but as any sex addict will tell you, the obsessive compulsion to experience romantic feelings, have sex, and make conquests is usually masking other buried problems.

Our society is so crazed about the issue of sex, our language overflows with crude, lewd, and strange words to describe doing it and not doing it. It's like the Eskimos and their many words for snow. Language is the carrier of culture, and we can learn a lot about our attitudes and beliefs by studying the words we use to talk about and describe celibacy and sex.

CELIBACY	SEX
spinster	hussy
old maid	whore
chastity	lust
pure	fornicator
frigid	hot
repressed	fuck

dried up	juicy
virtuous	hitting it
homosexual	homosexual
wimpy	screw
sissy	booty call
impotent	wild thing
sterile	getting some
good	bad
prude	knocking boots
bitch	bitch

Not to mention all the names we give to our body parts!

If you're not in a committed, monogamous, satisfying love relationship, there are lots of good reasons to practice celibacy.

HORMONAL PEACE. Remember PMS? The cramps, bloating, irritation, and general craziness? When our hormones are out of whack, we feel miserable.

One of the most common arguments against celibacy is that it's unnatural to deny the sex drive. Believe it or not, the physical feelings of sexual urgency calm down after a few months of no sex, though there may still be mental and emotional issues to work through. Dr. Winnifred Cutler, author of *Love Cycles: The Science of Intimacy,* says that unless a woman is having regular sex at least once a week, it's best for her to remain celibate. Sporadic bursts of sexual activity disrupt estrogen levels and fertility cycles. Cutler writes, "Biology seems to favor the woman who is slow to consider sexual congress; the woman who waits until she really knows her partner. . . . Until a woman meets such a man and gets to know him, celibacy preserves her hormonal system and her health."

Most important, a term of celibacy can offer a woman a physical rest and healing from vaginal soreness, yeast infections, and other sexually related problems. And sensual celibacy is 100 percent effective against sexually transmitted diseases.

EMOTIONAL HEALTH. Sensual celibacy gives a woman permission to focus on herself. Rebounding from a failed relationship only aggravates the pain. Time out from romantic involvements can help heal a broken heart and old wounds and give you a chance to gain new healthy perspectives on love, sex, men, and other relationship issues.

*H*ARRIET [LERNER, AUTHOR OF *THE DANCE OF ANGER*] MADE ME REALIZE THAT I HAD A TENDENCY TO PUT MORE SCRUTINY AND CARE AND CONCERN INTO PICKING A MELON FOR ONE FRUIT SALAD THAN I WOULD PUT INTO CHOOSING A BOYFRIEND FOR THE NEXT FIVE YEARS.

—MOLLIE KATZEN, AU-THOR OF *THE MOOSE-WOOD COOKBOOK*

CREATIVITY BOOST. When I talk to women about my most productive period of celibacy during which I wrote a book, worked a full-time job, started a company, and raised two children, I say, "What else did I have to do? I wasn't having sex!" A relationship in which sex is involved can be totally consuming, and when there is no relationship, no sex, you feel as if you have a lot of time on your hands.

One of the most satisfying benefits to solo time is the increased opportunity for creative expression. Write a poem, start a new business venture, design a dress—this is the best time to express yourself.

SPIRITUAL EXPANSION. No matter what your religion, faith, or belief system, the Sensual Celibacy Program will enable you to deepen your spiritual walk. Just when you thought you couldn't survive another lonely night, spiritual strengths such as courage, inner peace, patience, gratitude, forgiveness, and many others begin to take over the feelings of loneliness and desperation. The Program is adaptable to any faith or belief system.

PERFECT CONTRACEPTION. Women who have sex can get pregnant. Men who have sex don't get pregnant. You knew that already? Well, did you know that some men who impregnate women leave them? Celibacy is the sensible, practical choice of women of childbearing age.

My experiences have taught me the hard way that abstaining from sex until marriage is the only reasonable choice I personally can make. After what I've been through over the past few years, I'll never be able to fully trust a man's verbal commitment to marry me unless we're walking down the aisle. The fathers of my children both said they wanted to marry me. Both walked out on me while I was still pregnant. The discipline of celibacy has taught me to listen to what men say, watch what they do—*over time*—then make a decision.

GREATER INTIMACY. Whether involved in a romantic love relationship or a platonic one, women and men practicing sensual celibacy have the golden opportunity to get to know each other on deeper, more meaningful levels. Who knows? With sex tabled for the moment, maybe men and women can finally begin to approach a new, more loving age of effective communication, friendship, mutual respect, and understanding. And before you say "yeah, right," I challenge you to give it a try. Sex is so powerful that often we cannot hear what our partner is saying or see what he is really doing until it is too late. For women and men in the throes of infatuation, a practice of celibacy during the first few months will help a couple truly get to know one another and deepen their intimacy.

The Sensual Celibacy Program is for passionate, juicy, sexy, sassy women who have become celibate, temporarily or permanently, through choice or by "force." You may be waiting for Mr. Right, or abstaining for health reasons, grief, depression, or religious belief. Or maybe you're just tired and need time to regroup. This book gives you a nod and a blessing you may not get from family, friends, or society, with its harsh, intolerant, judgmental, prejudicial notions about celibacy and the women and men who practice it from time to time. You'll receive some useful tips and guidance on ways to make your practice of celibacy joyful, fulfilling, and fun. I hope you'll come away with a stronger acceptance of yourself.

The Program is also for those women who may be straddling the fence. Should you or shouldn't you practice celibacy at this time in your life? This book looks at the practice without the judgmentalism of religious dogma. Celibacy (and virginity) has nothing to do with issues of purity and chastity and more to do with practicality. It is not practical to have sex with a man, hoping that love and marriage will follow. It is not practical to have sex with a man you barely know. It is not practical to use sex to get to know a man. It is not practical to use sex to achieve instant intimacy. It is not practical to use sex to try and keep a man. It is not practical to engage in sexual relations with a man just because it feels good. It is not practical to use sex to lure a man away from another woman (if it happens to her, it could happen to you).

How many women do you know can have sex with no emotional connection? They do exist, but I don't think they're the norm. Sex is a bonding activity for most women. It makes us love and long for a man. When we have sex before a relationship has had the time and the opportunity to gel, we feel attached to a stranger who may or may not feel a similar connection. We are often left feeling anxious. (Will he call again? Will he respect me in the morning? Am I pregnant? Did I catch anything? Is he seeing someone else? Is he bisexual or gay?) Given all the unknowns in the early stages of a relationship, it is not practical to have sex until love and mutual trust (and for me, marriage) have been established. And that takes time.

If you're at the moment of truth in your relationship, and you're feeling that old, familiar tug in the lower regions, wait a minute and read *Sensual Celibacy* first. You're full of wonderful feelings and emotions right now, but I urge you to think through your decision. Don't allow yourself to be pressured. It may be the hardest thing you've ever done, but do this for yourself. It may be the right time to move into a sexual phase of the relationship, but it may not be. Allow yourself the time to figure it out honestly. Only you can decide what's right for you.

Finally, *Sensual Celibacy* is for tolerant, open-minded, sexually active women (and men) who want to understand the lifestyle and the emotional issues associated with celibacy in order to give support to friends and family who have made the decision to abstain from sex.

This book seeks to help women make their practice of celibacy a satisfying, productive, even joyful experience. I aim to prove, beyond a shadow of a doubt, that a woman practicing celibacy can still wear her miniskirts, bustiers, and lingerie with pride. She does not have to deny her sexiness or passion for life. It's time celibacy was brought out of the closet because nearly every woman (and man, quiet as it's kept) will close up shop at some point for some time in her life. Let's honor the decision to practice celibacy, advocate for its social acceptance as a legitimate, healthy lifestyle, and praise the courageous women (and men) who have dared to practice celibacy in the face of tremendous opposition.

CHAPTER ONE

Celibacy: Feast or Famine?

Q: Why did the chicken cross the road?
A: Because the grass looked greener on the other side.

There are two types of women in the world: Those who are having sex, and those who aren't. Over the years, as I was evolving this crude philosophy of women's sexuality, I came to another conclusion: Sexually active women are happy, satisfied, and fulfilled, while celibate women are miserable, pathetic wrecks, crying all the time.

It was a classic case of projection—me projecting my neurosis onto the entire world of women. It never occurred to me that celibate women could be happy, too. There's a danger in trying to oversimplify a complicated psychological and behavioral dynamic such as women's sexuality into neat black-and-white categories. If the world of women is composed of the sexually active and the sexually inactive as well as those who are in relationships and those who aren't, then we've just muddled up the stew quite a bit. Overlay those categories of women with needs, hopes, desires, wishes, dreams, emotional baggage, physical health, lifestyle choices, media manipulation, and societal expectations, and we have a nearly infinite variety of permutations and combinations, shades and shadows of sexual activity and celibacy. One woman's celibate practice may not be considered celibacy by another. One married woman's sexual involvement may not appear so holy to a single woman.

My earliest impressions of celibacy and sex came from the church I belonged to for the first eighteen years of my life. The women I categorized as not getting any were usually the church "nurses," uniformed in white polyester dresses, cheap wigs, and with a hospital smell. Women on the usher board might be married (and thus getting some), but usually they were widowed, lonely, older women with only themselves to keep each other company. They were the "spinsters" and the widows, who, after service, went back to bleak one-room kitchenettes that smelled like disinfectant. The younger women in their care came to church sans makeup, jewelry, and cute clothes. Their stockings were thick and dark, and their dresses hung about their bodies like laundry bags. Many were pretty, but their quiet, long-suffering, apolo-

CELIBACY IS HEREDITARY. IF YOUR PARENTS DIDN'T HAVE SEX, THE CHANCES ARE YOU WON'T HAVE SEX.
—ANONYMOUS

getic expressions dulled them. These poor souls would never get none as long as the spinsters and widows were in charge.

As for the married women, it was hard to imagine them getting any either. They seemed so somber and self-righteous, I couldn't picture them frolicking on the beach with some fine specimen of a man. They probably wanted to, but because they were stuck with the men they had, they were resigned to perfunctory, if any, sex. Their polyester dresses came in brown, black, navy, and forest green. Many wore fur coats and drove to church in old Cadillacs. Their flowered pillbox hats may have made them look respectable, but it was clear to me that their lives were drab, monotonous, and ordinary.

The women I categorized as "getting some," on the other hand, were single, glamorous, and smelled good. There was a constant aura of excitement and sin about them. They wore cheap mink stoles, lots of gaudy jewelry, smelled like cheap cologne, and their nails were long and red. They wore big, wild church hats atop their big, curly wigs. Their hips and breasts were conspicuous, and they walked with an exaggerated sway. Short, skinny men, fedoras in hand, would sit obediently next to them in the front pew. They, apparently, were the only women who could get a man to come to church.

Of course I couldn't possibly have known who was sexually active or who wasn't. The point is, somehow these perceptions around womanhood, femininity, and sex (or the lack thereof) developed early and subconsciously. I never consciously articulated my impressions as I grew up, but as I think back, I developed my perceptions about the women in my church based on how they smelled, felt, talked, and looked.

Even though I've grown in my understanding of women's sexuality, I must admit to some residual judgmentalism. I guess a woman's level of sexual involvement, or how much she is able to enjoy sex, by how she looks, smells, and feels when she hugs. If she hugs long and hard and smashes you with her breasts, she's tossing big salad. Women who have a live-and-let-live attitude about life are sexually satisfied or happy with their singleness. Women who are rigid and dogmatic in their beliefs (religious, political, or social) aren't getting any, or they aren't happy with what they're getting. Their hugs are perfunctory and cold, if they hug at all.

The road to maturity has been a long one, with fables marking the forks in the road: turn left to sanity, right to fantasyland. Given a choice between hard-core reality and fantasy, I always chose to believe in the impossible. The fables told to the girls of my generation demanded a suspension of disbelief. Take Sleeping Beauty. She was, for all intents and purposes, dead until a man resurrected her. She had no life until a godlike man breathed life into her body with a kiss. The prince rescued Cinderella from her bitchy "spinster" stepmother and stepsisters. The women of fables were never really whole until a man, a prince, transformed them into full-fledged women, envied and adored by society. That's what we want, we women, we sexual, romantic, social women. None of us witnessed in the lives of the adults we knew the romantic utopias dreamed up by those authors, but we wanted the illusion so bad we committed mind, body, and soul to the pursuit of love and romance.

When the 1960s sexual revolution stood America on its puritan head, I was still a girl and in the romance, fantasy mind-set. Sex for sex's sake just didn't appeal to my delicate, sensitive temperament, which no doubt was further complicated by my strict Christian upbringing. Yet I felt sucked into the flow by an undertow not of my own making. I was a late bloomer by the standards of the day: I was a college freshman when I finally said yes to sex. My first experience wasn't great, in fact it was pretty gloomy, but at least I was doing it and I was in love and I could finally hold my head up high in society. I had a man. Sort of.

For the next fifteen years, this would prove to be the pattern of my life: compelled to say yes to sex by the social current, but guilt-ridden because of church teachings that forbade premarital sex. I was full of fear—fear of pregnancy, sexually transmitted diseases, abandonment—but still saying yes. Anything could, and sometimes did, happen. Feeling that sex and love were meant to go together, I loved in order to have sex. Or did I have sex in order to have love? So much confusion, so much pain.

Ironically, my autobiography of sex is really about how I made a truce with celibacy. I had to. I've been single more than I've been in a couple. I've been celibate much more often than I've been sexually active. I was too scared to sleep around. I saw Looking for Mr. Goodbar. Hell and damnation themes were still burning in my subconscious. Given my never-ending desire for love and happiness with a man and my need to feel comfortable within society, celibacy and I have been uneasy partners.

Driven by the need for relationship magic and social acceptance, my choices in men were usually made in desperation. My shaky faith was dealt a further blow with the release of those horrible statistics that declared single women of a certain age had a better chance of getting attacked by a terrorist than getting married.

I asked myself, What's a Libra-born woman to do? They say Librans invented codependency. Maybe so, but the world could learn a thing or two from us natural born lovers. We know that a committed, intimate partnership can meet many emotional needs. Yet what we need to learn is how to survive the times when we're not in a relationship. This is our greatest challenge and, thus, our greatest opportunity for personal growth.

Women fear being labeled celibate, and so the euphemisms abound. We're "in between relationships" or "taking a break." Ironically, prior to the 1960s, women were expected to be "virtuous," that is, virgins or celibate outside of marriage. Today, in the secular realm, celibacy is a taboo subject. It is more acceptable for a gay man to admit he's gay than for a person practicing celibacy to come out of the closet.

Very few celebrities will admit to a celibate lifestyle because their success depends on their sex appeal—as if a celibate lifestyle and sex appeal cannot coexist in the same soul-body. The few brave souls who have made public declarations of their celibacy have been ridiculed and aligned with the radical Christian right. Heaven help them if they fall off the wagon or decide to become sexually active like Brooke Shields did. Such a smug public when it comes to this issue!

Celibate women are made to feel that somehow they are not "all woman," and celibate men are labeled gay, wimpy, or emotionally unbalanced. According to society, something's wrong with you if you're not having sex. The secret is, *nearly everyone will experience periods of celibacy at some point in their lives.* We all know this, yet we pretend that we're constantly sexually active. We wink, we smile mysteriously, but it's all a sorry pretense. We are less than honest when it comes to the celibate times in our lives, but we shout to the hills when we're sexually active!

All this dishonesty and contradictions in values fuel our desperation to try and find relief. Celibacy often comes into our lives so that we can sort out old, destructive patterns in relationships that we've been repeating over and over. We should welcome it, yet we run away from it. A hasty exit from celibacy will just about guarantee a repeat of the patterns and problems. When celibate periods are used to heal and grow, then we stand a better chance of not only discovering ourselves but finding and maintaining a satisfying love relationship.

> SENSUALITY IS COMPLICATED. LOVE IS INTRICATE. AND THE FLESH IS SWEET, BUT I NO LONGER MISTAKE IT FOR THE WHOLE THING.
> —CHRIS CHASE

Lest anyone get the wrong idea, let me clearly state here and now that I am not advocating celibacy over relationships. In fact my own biggest challenge is to not think about my solitude times as a waiting period, i.e., waiting for my mate to knock on my door. What I am advocating is women taking charge of their inevitable periods of celibacy in a positive way so that when relationship opportunities arise, their minds will be clear and their hearts will be healed enough to make intelligent decisions.

For example, if you're committed to working with the poor and your current love interest is a money-hungry tightwad, then you might need to reconsider this entanglement. If you're a devoted single mother of two and the object of your obsession can't stand kids, this might be a bad match. It doesn't matter how sexy the man is, if his life goals and values don't resonate with yours, you're looking at trouble.

Some women will say that even though they know their relationship is doomed, they're going to treat themselves to sex just because it feels good. They're going to wait on their soul mate while they're having sex with this other guy. Does this make sense? Is this practical? I think not! They claim they can handle uncommitted sex for sex's sake. I've got two things to say to that:

1. Can you really be so objective and detached from a man who has put his *penis* inside your *vagina,* for heaven's sake?

2. If your relationship goal is marriage or a long-term commitment, why risk the fulfillment of your dream by being involved in a relationship that you know is going nowhere? You have to sweep the house clean before you can move in new furniture.

After a sexual escapade, most women I know will continue to think and talk about the man. He penetrated her body, made an offering at her holy of holies, and now he is in her heart. He's all she can think about, and she waits by the phone for his call. Sexual involvement is good in marriages and long-term commitments because the goal is a healthy interdependency. The bonding that occurs during sex is a good thing—under the right circumstances. Relationships don't work if each partner is thinking of self and is being stingy with self. Premature sex in an as yet untried, new relationship, however, can have a devastating effect on a woman's heart, especially if all does not go well.

Yet, time and again, we women have sex before we're ready. Why? One reason is that celibacy forces us to deal with the self, which can be a scary thing. The quiet of solitude is threatening. The mirror's reflection haunts us. Some of us use the drama of relationships to hide from ourselves.

Social shame also drives us to make sexual decisions based on desperation. According to society, celibacy negates the sugar and spice that make a woman feminine. Sexual involvement validates her womanhood. "I have a man" is the saddest phrase spoken on TV talk shows today. It is usually spoken defensively, defiantly, and as a last resort to maintain some self-respect on national TV. When women say "I have a man," it's as if the essence of a woman's femininity and attractiveness has been validated. Just once I'd like a woman who's been put on the spot to say "It doesn't matter whether I've got a man or not. I'm a good woman. I'm a beautiful woman. I don't need a relationship to validate my femininity."

We are sexual beings, there's no denying that. Sex feels good. Even newborns touch themselves with pleasure. To create life, we must have sex. However, we are not animals. We're not at the mercy of instinct. We have minds, we can think. The sexual urge is powerful, but our minds are more so. But as powerful as our minds are, can they withstand the conspiracy of biology, societal expectations, and media manipulations? Sex surrounds us and teases us every day. On a daily basis we are penetrated by sexual images and themes in magazines, television, books, film, videos, and the Internet, and we orgasm every time we spend our dollars and time on these media products.

Speaking of the Internet, sex sells like crazy online. For a few bucks, you can have cybersex in chatrooms or look at pornography. Many special-interest groups have been expressing outrage and shock at the pornography that proliferates online. I don't like it either, but mess with online porn and you're messing with the First Amendment. I'm just sorry that celibacy is not an equally popular Internet topic. However, I'm not surprised. Online activities in the fourth dimension mirror the attitudes and behaviors in the physical third dimension. If the most outspoken advocates of sex are repressed about celibacy in the third dimension, then we will see that same attitude online. Not until society changes its mind about celibacy will there be a change in the fourth dimension.

I think that time is now. We're headed for a new millennium, a new day! It's time we destroyed the idea of the celibate woman as a cold, frigid fish and celibacy as a dry, famine time. Women practicing celibacy for a time are not "spinsters" or "old maids" or "dried up." We are juicy and self-determining and, dare I say, *sexy!* Why must so much dryness and death be associated with celibacy when the time offers so much opportunity for growth and fulfillment?

Practicing celibacy for self-determined periods of time forces us to honestly examine our attitudes around womanhood and femininity. Not only does sensual celibacy allow us to redefine old concepts in more life-affirming ways, it requires that we embrace our womanhood and femininity as individuals and not relative to someone else.

The best-kept secret in America today is the widespread practice of celibacy by people who are too intimidated to come out of the closet. It is more socially acceptable for women to admit they're celibate than men. However, the subject is often difficult for both women and men to discuss.

Graham Masterton notes in *Single, Wild, Sexy . . . and Safe* that "nobody has ever undertaken any serious research on the subject." Masters and Johnson, Janus, Kinsey, the University of Chicago, and mainstream women's magazines have all given a passing glance at celibacy *in context of* sexual practice, rather than studying it as a legitimate lifestyle choice in its own right. The implication is that celibacy is a sexual aberration. In fact, it is listed among the weird and unusual in the *Encyclopedia of Un-*

usual Sex Practices! But as we all know (even though we may not want to discuss it), we will all practice celibacy at some point in our lives, whether single or married, young or old, female or male.

Shere Hite's *Women and Love* is one of the very few studies to attempt to present a picture of celibacy in America. Although the main focus of this study is sex, we can still get a clue as to what's going on in the single beds. Hite's *Women and Love* is the final installment of a three-part report on women's sexuality. Fifteen thousand American women and men were surveyed between 1972 and 1986. Of the thousands of women interviewed,

*A*CCORDING TO A STUDY BY THE UNIVERSITY OF CHICAGO'S NATIONAL OPINION RESEARCH CENTER, MORE THAN 80 PERCENT OF THOSE SURVEYED SAID THEY HAD ONLY ONE [SEXUAL] PARTNER OR NO PARTNER AT ALL IN THE PAST YEAR.

27 percent of women say they feel that so much "sex" is just not worth it. And "Celibacy" ("no intercourse") was chosen by 33 percent of single women at one time or another, for a period of at least six months after they had been sexual earlier in their lives; almost all praise it because of the chance it gives them *not* to be sexually involved—to take an emotional break, focus their energy on other things. (Hite, p. 221)

If Hite's data is statistically sound, and her methodology suggests that it is, then a significant portion of the female population, fully *one-third of American women* (and that number may be low), are practicing celibacy at any given time, despite society's aversion to it. Furthermore, given the increased fear around sexually transmitted diseases in the 90s, it's safe to say that the number is probably higher today than when Hite conducted the study. Regardless, 33 percent of the population rates as a bona fide trend, not simply a fad. *Celibacy is a growing underground movement among American women.*

The Sensual Celibacy Program is a tool that promises to revolutionize women's approach to the sex-free times in their lives. No more beating the flesh into submission, no more chastity belts. Sensual celibacy acknowledges that as grown, adult women with common sense, strength, intelligence, emotional maturity, and courage, we can discipline our own selves. We can decide for ourselves when or if to begin or end a term of celibacy. We will no longer accept societal attitudes and prescriptions that drain us of energy, life, self-worth, and self-acceptance. We will decide for ourselves how we feel about the lifestyle we have chosen.

Keep a Sensual Celibacy Journal

Decision and self-determination are the keys to the practice of sensual celibacy. Women are notorious for being people pleasers. This trait of ours often keeps us saying yes to sex even when intercourse is not in our best interests. But first, you must understand your own attitudes about your sexuality. In-depth counseling may be required to get to the root of your behavior, but for now, the following self-assessment can help you begin to think about some of your attitudes and behaviors around sex and celibacy. I would strongly encourage you to keep a journal, taped or written, of your celibacy experiences—your successes, challenges, progress, setbacks. Maintaining a record of your feelings and experiences during this time is absolutely essential in helping you to measure your own progress. Keeping a journal is also very therapeutic. You can be totally honest about everything—no political correctness allowed! Just make sure you date each entry and keep your journal under lock and key!

No one but you has to know your answers. Here are some questions to ask yourself as you explore your attitudes toward sexuality:

+ Have you ever said yes to sex when you really wanted to say no? If yes, is this a pattern you've repeated over the years with different men? Why have you done this?

+ Have you ever experienced guilt feelings when you refused to have sex? If yes, do you think it is your responsibility to meet another's sexual needs?

+ Have you ever agreed to have sex, hoping that a love relationship, maybe even marriage, would come out of it?

✦ Do you ever allow yourself periods of celibacy (of any length) between relationships, or do you go from one relationship straight to another? Do your relationships overlap?

✦ In your practice of celibacy, how do you feel about yourself as a woman? How do you think your sexually active friends feel about your practice? How do you think you are perceived by society? Do you care?

✦ If you are currently celibate, do you think you were forced into the practice, or did you decide to become celibate?

✦ Have you ever had sex when you were physically ill? If yes, why did you do that? Have you ever had sex with a man who was physically ill? If yes, why did you do that?

✦ Do you ever feel as if you have to defend your celibacy practice to family and friends?

✦ Think of the celibate people you have known. What were your impressions about them?

✦ Do you have a support system that you can depend on to help you through the rough times?

✦ Do you ever discuss celibacy with your children as a smart choice? Do you expect them to remain virgins until marriage, or at least adulthood, or are you "realistic" and tell them to practice safe sex?

✦ Do your children get to know every man you get involved with?

There are no right or wrong answers. The purpose of this self-assessment is to get you off automatic ("I feel, therefore I have sex") and reclaim responsibility for your sexuality and behavior.

If you have children, the last two questions are really important. My personal goal with my own two children is to cancel the curse on women that has haunted my family for generations. The weaknesses of my foremothers were definitely passed on to me. Fortunately, my sisters, cousins, and I are growing in our awareness of the magnitude of the curse, and we're doing what we can to neutralize and lessen its effects on our daughters and sons. We're talking to them openly and honestly about love, sex, relationships, and marriage. We not only present virginity as a viable alternative to sex before marriage, we expect it of them. We've got to raise our expectations. Don't just accept safe sex—go for total abstinence.

We'll talk more about this later, but let me say just this much right now: If you are a parent, your children are watching every move you make. They're listening to everything you say, even when you think they've tuned you out. You are the primary role model for your children. If they see you with many different men, they're getting a specific message. You can't expect them to do as you say but not as you do. If you want them to have self-respect for their bodies, then you will have to demonstrate self-respect for your body: from what you eat, to how you take care of your body and your health, to abstaining from casual sex if you are single.

Another important element of your journal will be your "celibacy timeline." Don't worry about creating one right now. When we work through the first step of the program, I'll take you through the process. For right now, though, I want to share my own timeline with you.

Celibacy is an opportunity to raise the frequency of your life. It is the time for fine-tuning values that are life-affirming and self-empowering. "I'm not a nun!" you may object. Neither am I. I am not perfect. I slip up. I have fallen off the wagon. And I've learned to forgive myself and keep moving forward. I continue to try, and with time I've gotten better at my celibacy practice.

What happens when you don't practice sensual celibacy? Sexual energy has to be channeled in some way—some of us resort to alcohol and drug abuse, overeating, excessive masturbation, compulsive spending, and the final resort, unhealthy sexual affairs. Some of us do these things because we're sexually addicted, a clinical problem that deserves immediate treatment. I believe most of us are just earthy women, and it's for this group that the book is written. The Sensual Celibacy Program is about making your life so big that the excess sexual energy you may feel from time to time becomes less and less of a problem.

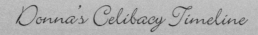

Donna's Celibacy Timeline

PERIOD 1:	12/83–4/85
PERIOD 2:	8/85–2/87
PERIOD 3:	8/88–4/92
PERIOD 4:	3/93–10/93
PERIOD 5:	3/94–7/96
PERIOD 6:	12/96–PRESENT

Periods defined here as celibate are based on Shere Hite's six-month guideline, i.e., you're celibate if you've not had intercourse for six months or more. These dates are rough estimates but help to organize my celibate periods from my divorce in 1983 to the present for the purposes of this book. Also, in the interest of accurate reporting (more or less), I fell off the wagon a couple of times during Periods 1 through 3, so in the classic sense, they were not true periods of celibacy. I include them here because 98 percent of those times I was not in a relationship. By the time I got to Period 4, however, I had gotten the hang of celibacy. No slipups!

CHAPTER TWO

The Sensual Celibacy Program

Celibacy is not a penance or a punishment. It represents an active choice, not a passive position.

—WINNIFRED B. CUTLER, PH.D.,
Love Cycles: The Science of Intimacy

◆ ◆ ◆

Remember Dr. Elisabeth Kübler-Ross's five stages of dying: denial, anger, bargaining, depression, and acceptance? From the end of a relationship through the period of celibacy, that's how many of us progress through this experience. In *Celibate Wives: Breaking the Silence,* authors Joan Avna and Diana Waltz report that married women who unwillingly become celibate also experience these five stages of dying. Arguably, celibacy in marriage might be the hardest type of all to manage. Single women expect the occasional vacation from sex. Nuns willingly forgo sex as part of their vocation. When we get married, however, the expectation to have sex with your husband is a given. The authors found that the reasons for a celibate marriage were many, including mismatched or low sex drives, abuse, infidelity, illness, and loss of respect. About 50 percent of the women chose to become celibate; the balance were forced into it against their wishes.

Although our needs and issues are different, single and married women who find themselves celibate share the grief experience—even those of us for whom celibacy is a welcome relief. Because our feminine identities are so tied up into whether or not we're sexually involved, the sudden or gradual removal of sex from our lives can call our identities as women into question. The loss of love and physical intimacy can at times seem unbearable. The social stigma can cause great shame. While this book addresses the needs of single women, Avna's and Waltz's insights into the emotional lives of celibate wives and their application of Kübler-Ross's framework to the grief experienced by celibate wives can guide us in understanding the stages many, if not most, single celibate women will go through.

DENIAL. "This can't be happening to me" best describes the emotional picture of this stage. "Denial helps you postpone the truth about your life" (Avna and Waltz, p. 44). The unreality of this period may be so overwhelming that you simply cannot handle it emotionally just yet. But according to Avna and Waltz, denial usually "crumbles piece by piece." Most women I know (including me) process through this period by incessantly discussing how bad an ex was. He did this, he did that. While the relationship was going strong, we focused on the good times; during denial, we focus on the bad. By focusing on our ex's bad behaviors, we deny our own contributions to the demise of the relationship. Denial is accompanied by a lot of pain, a lot of grieving.

ANGER. Then we get *pissed off.* This is the stage when my women friends start plotting to blow up property, specifically their ex's. I have had my moments too. After one especially difficult breakup, I fantasized day and night about tearing up his nice suits, bombing his car, and smashing all the windows in his house. I'm really a slow burn, so the intensity of my anger surprised me. Years later when I saw the movie version of *Waiting to Exhale,* I have to admit, I couldn't help smiling when Angela Bassett's character went berserk, destroying the property of her cheating, no-good husband.

I don't recommend staying in this stage forever, but there is an energizing force to righteous anger. In the denial stage, the grief and sorrow can drain you of all your energy, but anger—now that's an emotion that will kick you out of bed in the morning.

BARGAINING. "If only I could lose the weight, I would find a mate." That's me! Now and then I still slip into bargaining! Deep down I know that finding that special man really has nothing to do with how many pounds I need to lose, but this kind of mental dickering helps me believe that I can control the outcome of my situation. How many of us bargain with God or ourselves, as if our "predicament" was some sort of marketplace in which circumstance could be sold away for a promise? "Bargaining offers hope that your celibacy is not permanent, that you can still change or fix it and your life will be better" (Avna and Waltz, p. 59).

DEPRESSION. "Why me?" is the anguished cry of the depressed celibate woman. You're a good woman. You're kind to animals and the elderly. The fairness of your situation eludes you, especially when you know some royal witches who have men falling all over them. What are you doing wrong?

Nothing. In fact, by holding out for your true soul mate, you're doing everything right. What makes life difficult for the single celibate woman is that there is so little support for her practice. There are few, if any, attractive, sexy celibate role models on TV or film. As we've said before, celibacy is ridiculed by the general society. Why should you feel like a party when your current lifestyle is perceived as abnormal by so many people? Many women and men practicing celibacy feel they must keep that part of their lives secret and hidden away in the closet. We pay in the long run, however, because to mask such an important aspect of our lives is to deny our essential selves. You begin to heal from depression when you begin to live life authentically.

It's Patty who chose a life of celibacy. Selma simply had celibacy thrust upon her.

—MARGE SIMPSON, THE SIMPSONS

ACCEPTANCE. During Celibacy Periods 1 through 3 (see page 43), which was spread over nearly ten years of my life, accepting my situation was the hardest of the five stages to process through. The social shame and loneliness made me one desperate woman, and usually I would move directly from the depression stage straight to a relationship, which of course would be doomed from the very start. What made Celibacy Periods 5 and 6 so meaningful and productive, however, is that I *started out* with acceptance. I was so grateful for the opportunity to get my life together that I couldn't experience anything else but success.

Although in my earliest experiences with celibacy I did indeed feel like I was dying, I slowly discovered that I did not have to experience celibacy solely through these stages. Like everything else in life, I could choose to make the experience work for me. And so I did.

Let's find out where you are in the five stages. The following questions have been designed to help you assess not only where you are, but where you should be heading. Use your sensual celibacy journal, if you're keeping one, or get out some sheets of paper, and expand on any question that strikes you. There's no rating system here, because only you can determine where you are emotionally.

Denial

+ Despite every indication to the contrary, are you still hoping for a reconciliation with your ex-boyfriend or -husband?

+ Do you continue to call your ex for concocted reasons ("I just wanted to see how you were doing")?

+ Do you purposefully leave items behind so that you have a reason to see your ex again ("Did I leave my CD over at your house? Can I come get it?")?

+ Do you continue to have sex with your ex even though the relationship is over?

+ How long have you been legally separated from your husband? Years?

+ Are you consciously practicing a healthy celibacy, or are you not having sex by default (i.e., you haven't made a love connection)?

+ Is fear of intimacy the true reason for this no-sex time?

+ Are you like Dick Tracy, spying on your ex? Why are you spying on him when the relationship is over?

+ Do you obsessively think about your ex? When the phone rings, do you pray it's him?

+ Do you still call your ex just to say "hi," even though he's told you he doesn't want to talk to you anymore?

+ Since your breakup with your ex, have you been rebounding with other men?

Anger

+ Do you fantasize about blowing up your ex's car, shredding his clothes, doing him physical harm? Do you enjoy this fantasy?

+ This is a combination denial/anger issue: Are you snapping at your children, coworkers—everyone else but the true object of your anger, your ex?

+ Have you hit anyone in anger?

+ Have you threatened to physically harm your ex?

Bargaining

+ Do you think that losing five pounds might make your ex change his mind?

+ Do you use time to bargain with yourself ("I'll wait two months, and then I know I'll have a new relationship")?

+ Have you negotiated a deal with the Supreme Being to join church/temple/mosque/synagogue upon receipt of a new boyfriend/husband?

+ When you heal from this broken heart, are you counting on love finding you?

+ Do you bargain with the fates over the idea that when you're not looking for love, love will appear? Are you, thus, determined to not look for love in order to get love?

Depression

+ Do you spend more time in the bed than on your feet?

+ Have you felt so sad that you've had to call in sick to work?

+ Have you lost/gained weight?

+ Have you completely lost all desire for sex?

+ Are you drinking excessively? Doing drugs?

+ Have you any emotional energy to spare for your children? Family and friends?

- Do you feel like you want to die sometimes?

- Do you watch too much TV?

- When was the last time you showered? Washed your hair?

- Do you feel tired all the time?

- Do you believe that you've suddenly become physically un-attractive?

- Are you ashamed to be without a man?

- Do you feel like a failure?

Acceptance

- Do you feel little but significant bursts of happiness for no reason?

- Are you able to live with an unknown future and still be happy?

- Do you have faith in your own abilities?

- Do you believe that you're physically attractive?

- Are you able to think positive thoughts about your ex?

- Do you love yourself unconditionally, despite your idiosyn-cracies and weaknesses?

- Are you now able to bless your former relationship for the lessons that you learned?

- Are you happy to be alive?

- Do you forgive your ex?

- Do you appreciate this time off from relationships and sex?

- Do you care what other people may have to say, positive or negative, about your singleness?

The first time I got celibacy right, Period 5, I was about thirty-five years old. I had two children, a full-time job, and a budding career as a writer. My life was difficult—how does one ever balance career and children? In addition, I was in a relationship that didn't satisfy me. He was a good man with a good heart, but the timing was not right for us. We drifted apart, and for the first time in my life, I chose celibacy. I sought it out; I put it on like a life jacket. Celibacy did not come and grab me by the throat as it had in the past. I eagerly, willingly entered into it and stayed happily put for about four years (minus one six-month relationship that included sex). During that time I got so much done I amazed even myself. I held down a demanding full-time job, started a company, wrote four books, and raised two children with the help of my wonderful, supportive family.

I was not occupied emotionally, mentally, or physically with a man. I was not cooking or cleaning for a man, nor was I worrying about whether or not a man was ever going to call me again, or leave me. I had plenty of time and opportunity to finally get to know myself and work on achieving some of my life-mission goals.

I also used the time to heal from old relationship wounds and destructive patterns. I still longed for marriage and love and romance, but my unswerving focus on my goals took the place of my man search, took the edge off my loneliness, and totally neutralized my old feelings of desperation.

For the first time in my life, I felt strong. Feelings of power and control caused me to totally reconsider my definitions of femininity and womanhood, which had their roots in church teachings. I had been programmed to believe that a woman's role is to support a man. Someone has to lead, and God appointed Man to serve in that capacity. Yet, in all the institutions in my community—churches, schools, families, social service organizations, businesses—women run everything. During the civil rights movement of the 1960s, men might have gotten all the media attention, but it was women who were cooking, cleaning, typing, filing, answering phones, organizing rallies—as well as

THE MOST EXCITING MEN IN MY LIFE HAVE BEEN THE MEN WHO HAVE NEVER TAKEN ME TO BED.

—EARTHA KITT

getting beaten and thrown in jail with the men. Men might be more visible, e.g., the pastor of a church, but women run the show.

But isn't this typical of woman's work in communities all across America? Feminists fought for such basic human rights as equal pay for equal work, and few can deny their valid contributions to the noble goals of justice and equality for all.

If I were to launch a feminist movement, however, I would protest, boycott, and sit in for *less* work, more siestas, and help around the house. After a day of working, cooking, cleaning, and raising children, what I really need is sleep. I would also lobby the medical establishment on conducting research to find out how men can start having the babies.

All women are stressed because so much of the workload falls on our shoulders. But we are stressed for another reason too. The pursuit of a relationship, or the attempt to try and keep one, can cause great anxiety. We women have a poverty and scarcity mentality when it comes to men. We don't think there are enough to go around, so we moan and scheme and long with all of our hearts for that one man who will make us happy. Too often we engage in sexual relations way before we should. We share men and even have affairs with married or otherwise engaged men.

So during this wondrous period of celibacy, I dared to envision a future relationship characterized by partnership, mutual sharing, respect, honesty, monogamy—and, of course, love. I used that period to redesign my life, my beliefs, and my values in any way that I wanted. I could throw out old ideas that no longer served me.

Carl Jung said that we all have male and female aspects. During Period 5, I felt as if my male side was coming out of hiding for the first time in my life. I had vision. I was seeking out and conquering new territories. I was confident and strong.

I have to admit, however, that I often missed the feminine me. My lacy panties had been replaced by boxer shorts. My emotions were developing muscles, and although I liked it, there were moments of discomfort. Feminine power I knew well. I knew how to bear the pain of childbirth and menstruation. I knew how to nurture and raise children. I had learned to trust the still, small voice within, i.e., my feminine intuition. But this penetration into the world in such a vigorous, aggressive way—it was as if some alien being had taken over. I was a force of nature. I began speaking up for myself. My personality in relationships up until that time was akin to a doormat. The new me no longer allowed herself to be stepped on. The old me avoided confrontations; I now clashed like a Titan. When I perceived that someone was mistreating me, I fought back. Today, the extremes are balancing themselves out. I am learning to be feminine and strong, nurturing and firm.

I believe in the Sensual Celibacy Program. I can't promise that you'll find the man of your dreams, but I can guarantee that you will become the woman that you've always known in your heart you could be. I wish I could say that the Program will replace Kübler-Ross's stages of dying, but realistically, some grief, anger, and depression will probably occur, especially if your entry into celibacy was traumatic. However, if you make the decision to become celibate and commit to using the Program as a guide, you will not be sorry.

The following steps are designed to help you matriculate through your term of celibacy safely, productively, and happily. They are listed here sequentially for clarity, but in practice, you'll probably want to work on some areas concurrently, while saving others for when you are emotionally ready. For the most part, that's okay. However, the first step really should go first.

Read through the steps with an open mind, then give them a try. The most important idea underlying all 10 steps is to learn to listen and trust the guidance you have within. The 10 steps of the Sensual Celibacy Program are:

1. Begin decisively

2. Know thy celibate self

3. Set, then pursue, goals

4. Heal your soul

5. Strengthen your celibacy practice

6. Mind your body

7. Get out of the house and mingle

8. Give men the benefit of the doubt

9. Model a healthy, happy celibate lifestyle

10. End intelligently and decisively

Notice that the Program takes you from *beginning* to *end* of your celibacy practice. That's right, hallelujah, there's an end in sight, there's a light at the end of that tunnel, there's a man a'coming! But not before you're ready. Lord knows we don't want to be celibate forever! Sensual celibacy is for women who want to be in a relationship and are willing to journey through this wild and fabulous wilderness experience until they are mentally, physically, emotionally, and spiritually ready to engage in the *big event*. As you use the Program to enhance your practice, you will be amazed at your growth and development. You might even begin to enjoy your own company so much that the final exit step could be cause for some anxiety! We'll talk more about that in chapter 12.

> WHAT DO I KNOW ABOUT SEX? I'M A MARRIED MAN.
>
> —TOM CLANCY

Sensual celibacy is definitely the road less traveled in America. Instant gratification characterizes our society, and consistently and deliberately saying no to something that is thrown in our faces every day takes courage, strength, and skill. The Sensual Celibacy Program offers skill-building exercises, self-esteem-boosting affirmations, guided imagery, meditations, and self-assessments.

There's no time like the present to get started. Beginning well is your first step to a healthy, productive, sensuous celibacy practice. Before you begin, a couple of guidelines: All exercises in this book have been designed to make your sexual time-out a productive and healing one. The guidelines can be used by women who are celibate or women who are currently sexually active but are planning for a period of celibacy. Answer the questions and do the exercises with as much honesty as you can muster. Don't worry about sounding pitiful or ashamed.

There's a highly popular self-help technique called "act as if." If you're poor and you want to be rich, act as if you're rich. If you're sad and want to be happy, act as if you're happy. The problem with "act as if" is that you're attempting to cover up problems that really need to be exposed to the light of your awareness. You can "act as if" all you want to, but I guarantee, if you don't deal with the root issues first, they're going to arise when you least want or expect them.

Don't be afraid of sorrow. Sorrow is a natural, healthy, normal response to setbacks. Let yourself experience it—or whatever you're feeling. Believe with all your heart that what you're feeling is a valid and necessary part of the healing process and this too will pass in its own time. *Just be honest with yourself.*

Many of us celibate women are like the walking wounded. Counseling is, of course, one of the best ways to process through grief. The Sensual Celibacy Program can easily be done in conjunction with your counseling sessions. Just make sure you let your therapist know what you're up to.

Now let's decide to become happy and sensually celibate—and that's no oxymoron!

AFFIRMATION: *I'll keep getting the same results if I keep doing the same old stuff. My mind is open to giving sensual celibacy a try.*

CHAPTER THREE

Step 1—
Begin Decisively

✦ ✦ ✦

You've just broken up with a man. Or maybe he abandoned you. Or maybe your beloved died. Or maybe you're recuperating from an illness. Or maybe you're sexually active but are considering celibacy. This can either be the best of times or the worst of times. It all depends on your attitude. How you enter into a period of celibacy can determine how productive this period will be.

Have you entered into celibacy reluctantly or deliberately? For many of us, being in a relationship is preferable to being alone. That's why celibacy can be so hard at first. Look, no woman *has* to be celibate. There is plenty of sex to go around, if that's all you want. No doubt you want more. You deserve more. Here's where the issue of *decision* enters into our enlightened approach. If you can begin to realize that no one forced you to become celibate, that you made this choice on your own, then you'll be able to accept it and move on to bigger and better things.

Before getting into this first step, answer the following questions. They will help you to start *thinking* about what you're going through and assess how well your values and behaviors around sex, relationships, and celibacy are serving you. Don't forget to record your answers in your journal.

Self-Assessment Exercise

If you are *considering celibacy,* meditate on the following questions:

✦ Why are you considering celibacy at this time?

✦ What has prevented you thus far from becoming celibate?

✦ What are your thoughts about celibacy? What are your thoughts about people who are celibate? Do you know anyone who is celibate? What are your thoughts about the person's practice of and attitude toward celibacy?

+ Are you considering breaking up with your current partner? Or are you considering celibacy while still in the relationship?

+ What do you need to do to make the final decision?

+ What frame of mind/emotional state do you need to reach to make the final decision?

+ If you're newly single, do you think you could decide to be celibate while still caring for and being sexually attracted to your partner?

+ How does the possibility of becoming celibate make you feel? (Note all that apply.) Afraid _____ Hopeful _____ Anxious _____ Proud _____ Defeated _____ Ashamed _____ Relieved _____ Angry _____ Morally Correct _____ Other _____

_____

If you are currently in a relationship but are considering becoming celibate, (1) you're planning a breakup with your partner/spouse, or (2) your mate is about to get a most interesting proposition. If you fall in the first group, your decision involves much more than simply not having sex for a while. You're about to sever a soul tie with a man with whom you share history. That's not easy. The steps of this Program can help you heal during this difficult period. If you belong to the second group, your situation is beyond the scope of this book. However, a friendly word of advice: You're not in the relationship by yourself. Talk to your mate about your desire, don't just announce it. More than likely, this will cause him some stress. He may get angry. Allow him his anger. No one gets into a relationship to become celibate, and your proposition might take him totally by surprise. A compromise might be to suggest a very brief period of abstinence. Counseling can help you both sort through all the issues.

If you are *currently celibate*, meditate on the following questions:

+ Why have you entered into celibacy? Do you feel you have entered by choice or by force?

✦ How long have you been celibate? Has it been too long, just enough time, or not enough time since you've had sex?

✦ How would you rate your sense of self-worth on a scale from 1 to 10? If your self-worth is low, does not having sex have anything to do with it?

✦ Are you currently dating? If not, would you like to date? What's preventing you from dating? If you are dating, are you ever tempted to waver from your commitment to your celibacy practice? What do you do to keep temptation at bay?

✦ What do you do about horniness? Loneliness?

✦ Is there a certain time of the day/week/month/year that's more difficult than others? Are holidays difficult for you? If so, how do you handle them?

✦ What are your thoughts about celibacy? What are your thoughts about people who are celibate? Do you know anyone who is celibate? What are your thoughts about the person's practice of and attitude toward celibacy? Is that person a good or bad role model?

✦ What kind of support system do you have? Are most of your friends single or married, sexually active or celibate? How happy are they with their situations?

✦ How does being celibate make you feel? (Note all that apply.) Afraid _____ Hopeful _____ Anxious _____ Proud _____ Defeated _____ Ashamed _____ Relieved _____ Angry _____ Morally Correct _____ Other _____

✦ If you still care for and/or are sexually attracted to your ex-mate/ex-spouse, are you ever tempted to waver from your commitment to celibacy and have sex with him? What are your thoughts? What are your feelings? What do you do to manage temptation?

✦ Did your ex quickly find a replacement for you? If yes, does this tempt you to rebound with another man?

◆ How strong/weak are you in your commitment to practice celibacy?

Obviously, there are many different permutations and combinations of situations that women bring to their relationships and celibacy practice, and not all can be dealt with here (e.g., married women who are celibate). Still, answering the above questions should help many women begin to make their practice of celibacy a conscious one. Awareness and empowerment are the goals. Don't use your answers to beat up on yourself. We all have areas that need improvement. We all have regrets, and anyone who has ever loved a man has done some crazy things. We've all been there. You're not alone. Use the self-knowledge to fuel your self-improvement plan (chapter 5).

BARBARA WALTERS: I DON'T NEED A MAN TO HAVE A GREAT TIME.

—*NATIONAL ENQUIRER* HEADLINE, JANUARY 21, 1997

RECONSTRUCT YOUR CELIBACY TIMELINE. At the end of chapter 1, I presented for your review a timeline of my celibacy periods since my divorce in 1983. What a grueling, tedious exercise! I mean, I absolutely hated doing it. It brought back all

*I*N THE ARTICLE, BARBARA IS QUOTED AS SAYING "SEX ISN'T ALL IT'S CRACKED UP TO BE" AND "I CAN DO IT ALL FOR MYSELF."

the old pains and boyfriends that I had buried long ago. Like many people, I tend to block out a lot of the bad stuff. I actually had to use my work résumé to help me remember.

The exercise did provide me with some crucial self-knowledge, however. Now I have a map that describes my relationship history and patterns, as well as my progress. For example, although in Period 2 I was as desperate as ever to snare a husband, I made significant progress in my spiritual development by deprogramming myself of the more negative and controlling aspects of church involvement. This period was critical in getting me to think about that age-old question, Who am I?

As I review my timeline I realize that I'm not so bad after all, and even though I haven't always realized it, my life is always being divinely guided.

What a blessing to finally become aware of the activity of my God in my life! Constructing the timeline may or may not be fun for you. Do it anyway, and don't fret if you don't get the dates exactly right. Approximates are fine.

I followed Shere Hite's six-month rule of celibacy, only including those periods that lasted six months or longer. If you cannot remember such a time, then write down any memorable times when you were not sexually involved with a man. This too will be helpful in understanding how past relationships and periods of celibacy have created the pattern that has led to your current situation.

Another piece of critical information that will emerge are the times when your celibacy was not "pure"—i.e., when you jumped off the wagon and did the wild thing. Those times are also important to note, as well as the reasons for the lapses.

I also discovered a pattern of relationship repeats—for example, the relationships following Periods 3 and 5 were with the same man, and there are a couple more. My new philosophy is this: Never look back! Keep moving forward! Repeat relationships just don't work for me.

I didn't include names and juicy situations in this published version, but you'll want to include all the gory details in your own journal.

MAKE A DECISION. What, no sex at all? Like Gloria Gaynor says, you will survive. Haven't you always? Besides, if it's your choice, you won't be alone forever. Granted, our society makes practicing celibacy about as difficult as swimming upstream. It wasn't always like this. In our not so distant past, a single woman was expected to practice celibacy or be labeled a whore. Issues of freedom and self-determination notwithstanding, there was social support for single women who abstained from sex. Also, there wasn't the complete pervasiveness of sexual images and themes in media. It's all a passionate women can do to keep her own raging hormones in check without men's jeans ads constantly titillating her.

Think of it this way: No sex for a while doesn't mean that you can't have a man in your life. In fact, the more the merrier! Now that sex has been put on hold for a moment, it's a great time to cultivate relationships with men and get to know them as individuals, not penis machines. All these "rules" about not approaching men—forget them. Make friends with men the same way you make friends with women. Just be your sweet, loving, sensual self!

Decide today to commit to a self-loving, productive celibacy practice. Not deciding is also making a decision. You give your power away to the fates when you fail to take responsibility for your life. Don't stay in limboland. Don't give your power up to whomever or whatever the winds blow your way. Decide right now to commit to a six-month term of celibacy. Six months is not an eternity. Aren't you worth this brief moment in time? Isn't your growth and development worth it?

Yes, self-improvement can occur while you are sexually active, especially if you receive support from your partner. The truth is, most of us will get involved with a man and totally forget about our self-improvement program. We forget what day of the week it is! Celibacy will give you at least six months of uninterrupted time to focus on yourself and no one else, and that is truly a gift.

Now that you've thought about your reasons for your celibacy practice and the way you've been managing your relationships, can you make a commitment to practice celibacy for a period of time? If you can, complete the contract below. If not, that's okay. Read on. I hope to make a case powerful enough to cause you to reconsider!

Notice that your Celibacy Promise has a line for a witness's signature. This is optional, but I would highly recommend having a trusted friend, counselor, or family member sign. Later in this chapter we'll talk about developing a support network, but for now, think about choosing as your witness someone who loves you, someone you can trust. This person should support and reinforce your commitment to practice celibacy for at least six months. She or he should help keep you honest. Also, make sure your witness reads this book from cover to cover, especially the parts about sensual celibacy as a *nonjudgmental, compassionate* practice. The last thing you need right now is someone making you feel ashamed or less than whole. Your witness should be firm but loving, honest but not critical or judgmental. Choose this person wisely.

BE GRATEFUL. For those of us who wanted a respite from sex, we're probably full of gratitude. However, if you've entered into celibacy

Sensual Celibacy Promise

I, _____, an unattached single woman, decide today to practice celibacy. I commit to a sensual practice that is gentle, loving, productive, and fun. My practice will build on my strengths and forgive my weaknesses.

Today's date is _____. I will not have sex for at least six months from today's date. Furthermore, if in six months I am not either married or in a committed, monogamous, loving relationship, I will not panic. I will continue to practice celibacy. I hereby announce today that my health and sanity are well worth the wait!

SIGNED: _____

WITNESSED BY: _____

under traumatic circumstances, if you hate the fact that you're celibate, it may be extremely difficult to feel grateful right now. Please, hear me out: An attitude of gratitude is absolutely essential to the success of your practice. A bitter attitude will only bring about bitter results.

For those of you already happy about your situation, here's a little meditation to say upon awakening and whenever you think of it throughout the day:

I am grateful for this golden opportunity alone to discover who I am and to improve myself.

Reluctant celibates can start out their day with this thought:

I have to be honest with myself. I don't feel grateful, but I believe with all my heart that all things are working together for my good right now. I have faith, and for that, I am grateful.

Developing the attitude of gratitude (especially when you don't feel grateful) is a skill that can be learned and a muscle that can be developed. Do an inventory of all the things in your life that are good. Make a daily practice of being thankful. ("Thank you, God, for health. Thank you for good family and friends. Thank you for my car. Thank you for pretty hair. Thank you for food and shelter.") Too often a state of celibacy becomes the overwhelming, dominant thought. We forget about all the wonderful things that are going well. Prayers of gratitude help women gain much needed perspective and are an excellent first step on the road to healing and self-discovery. Be thankful morning, noon, and night, and you'll be amazed at the difference in your attitude, your celibacy practice, and your life!

FORGIVE YOURSELF, FORGIVE OTHERS. Forgive yourself. Forgive your ex. One of the biggest obstacles to a successful celibacy practice is the inability to forgive. Like gratitude, forgiving is a skill and a muscle; it must be practiced and strengthened, even when you don't feel like it.

Forgiving yourself and your ex is an essential prerequisite to your healing. Your ability to forgive is for your benefit. You can harbor a grudge all you want, but I guarantee, while these angry feelings are eating away at your body, compromising your immune system, and making you sick physically and psychologically, the object of your anger is going on with his life.

For your own sake, meditate on the following until the ideas become truth for you:

I forgive myself. I love myself unconditionally. I forgive those who have hurt me. I may not feel like forgiving right now, but I forgive anyway. And So It Is.

Answer this question honestly: Are you more interested in being right or do you want to heal? Regardless of what was done to you, regardless of how justified your anger may be, the bottom line is that grudges only hurt you. Throughout your term of celibacy, you'll need to revisit forgiveness often.

GET A CHECKUP. Another important thing that you must do in this first stage: Go get a gynecological checkup. If you've had one or multiple partners, it makes no difference. While intercourse brings ecstasy, it can also bring disease. I heard a woman say once that there's more to the lowly yeast infection than meets the eye. Symbolically, that deep, yearning, incessant itch symbolizes love needs unfulfilled. Literally, yeast may not be yeast. It may be a lot more. Whether or not you have symptoms, get a thorough checkup. Sexually transmitted diseases are running rampant, and it only takes one episode of intercourse to catch something. Do yourself a favor and schedule an appointment with your gynecologist today.

TRUST THE PROCESS. Think about all the times that you were afraid of doing a thing because you didn't think you could do it but, lo and behold, you surprised yourself with a mighty accomplishment. If you go through the steps of the Sensual Celibacy Program as they have been described in this book, you will be amazed at how fulfilling your time alone will be. I hope that in the next few chapters I'm able to persuade you in the wisdom, beauty, and simplicity of the Program. The rest will be up to you. The fact that you are reading this book at all says a lot about your ability to take risks and about your adventurous spirit. You are a nonconformist in the best sense of the word.

If you watch the news every day, it's easy to lose faith in the benevolence of the universe, but don't give in to the moan and groan choirs, the pity parties, the miserables who love your company. Now that you've decided to commit to at least six months of abstaining from sex, you'll be amazed at the changes that'll take place in your life. Trust in the helpful forces in the universe to assist you in making this time the most productive, satisfying, and fun time you've ever had. Just be careful; you will get what you ask for!

DEVELOP A SUPPORT NETWORK. If you have a solid support network, great. You're one step ahead of the game. Even so, do a careful inventory of your friends. If there are any who drain you of your energy or even hint at any intolerance of your celibacy practice, get rid of them. They're dead weight.

Of course you can't control everyone who flows in and out of your life, but you can control who, in your personal, private times you choose to give your love and attention to. Choose your confidants wisely.

Talk to friends. Talk to a therapist, a minister, a trusted family member. Allow yourself time to grieve. Have the courage to let yourself feel the sorrow. I wish there was an easier way, but there's not. It's a law of nature—that from which you attempt escape will always come back to haunt you. You cannot escape trials and tribulations in life, and it is the mature woman who stands fast and refuses to run and hide in the bed of a stranger. Mature women, however, will talk out their needs, desires, and longings. Through talking we heal.

Mr. Right is now a guy who hasn't been laid in fifteen years.
—ELAYNE BOOSLER

Never underestimate the power of sisterhood. Seek out strong, compassionate, positive women who will allow you to rest your weary head on their shoulder. A good friend will hear your story over and over until you've gotten it out of your system. I don't know what I would have done without my sisters and women friends. We've all been down the same road a few times, and it's good to know that when I need them, they're there for me, as I am there for them. During my early flirtations with celibacy, I weathered the storms alone and was not nearly as successful as when, in the later periods, I turned to my sisters and, much later, my friends for support.

Now that you've signed the Celibacy Promise, how do you feel?

+ I'm excited!

+ I'm scared that committing to celibacy will send a message to men to stay away.

+ I'll wait and see.

To those of you who checked the first answer, Hurray! Whoopee! I'm excited for you because you're about to experience a great adventure that will change your life for the better.

To the women who checked the second answer, I understand your fear. I no longer agree with it, but I understand it. As you'll learn in chapter 10, you'll be amazed at the men who will be attracted to you. It all depends on your attitude.

And to the women from Missouri who checked the third answer, I can appreciate your wait and see attitude. I also appreciate your willingness to give the Program a try. Just keep an open mind!

AFFIRMATION: *Oh, happy day! I've made a decision that will change my life forever. I feel like dancing. I think I will! Also, a promise is a promise. I am a woman of my word!*

CHAPTER FOUR

Step 2—Know Thy Celibate Self

I want to be alone.

—Greta Garbo

There's nothing like a long vacation from sex to force the real issues to the table such as, Who am I? Who am I as a woman? What is the essence of my femininity? What is my life mission? What can I do to make this stint of celibacy happy and productive?

Adventure vacations have become quite popular with women seeking to raise the pitch of their lives. They allow women to access reserves of courage and endurance and pit their strength and wits against the elements. Women are climbing mountains, whitewater rafting, and hiking all over the world.

Think of this period of celibacy as an adventure vacation from sexual involvement. This adventure will motivate you to explore the deepest regions of your being, the farthest expanses of your consciousness. You will be tapping physical, emotional, mental, and spiritual resources that you never knew you had.

For many women, relationships can be like straitjackets restricting freedom of thought, word, and movement. Either we're catering to a man's ego at the expense of our own, or we're afraid of revealing too much of ourselves. Either way, our big, beautiful spirits can only stand so much suffocation, which may be one reason why your relationship didn't work out. You weren't being true to yourself. You were too focused on someone else.

Self-actualization is about becoming fully human. Too often in our relationships with men we compromise and give away this precious gift in order to keep the peace. Self-actualization can be a messy business, but boy, is it ever satisfying. There's such freedom in being who you are and not giving a damn what anyone else has to say about it! There may be trade-offs in the beginning. For example, as you grow too big for your cultural shell, you'll probably find that you and your friends no longer share the same interests. Don't be surprised if they begin to question your actions. They may stop calling altogether. That's why it's so important to build your support network with care.

Also, beware this law of the universe: Like attracts like. As you begin to change and grow, you'll find that you no longer enjoy the same type of man you dated in the past. Just be observant and keep recording your observations in your journal. The great adventure has only just begun!

Know Your Celibacy Type

Many of us go through celibacy as quickly as we can, without taking the time to think about our values, goals, and dreams as they relate to sex, relationships, and our celibacy practice. Because we are all so different, with our unique dreams, desires, needs, and emotional programming, women practice celibacy in a variety of ways. The following is my laywoman's mixed bag of categories and descriptions of some of the different types of celibates and celibacy practices.

PROFESSIONAL CELIBATES include nuns, monks, and priests. Sexual abstinence is required as part of their vocation.

RETIRED CELIBATES are individuals who have enjoyed sex in the past (or maybe not) and are now quite content to live without it. Maybe a spouse has died and the surviving partner does not wish to re-marry. This category might also include some seniors, as well as women who have chosen to permanently channel their energy into worthy causes or creative pursuits. Other Retired Celibates are former Serial Celibates (below) who never resolved their destructive relationship patterns and now are too bitter to want to try again.

SERIAL CELIBATES haven't fully reconciled themselves to a celibate lifestyle. There is something threatening and scary about singleness. While they may abstain fro a brief time, they're using the time alone to find a man (or woman) to fill the void. Often, they overlap relationships, that is, before a breakup occurs they already have someone else lined up. These patterns repeat time and again, providing little opportunity to heal past wounds and reflect on mistakes made in past relationships.

TECHNICAL CELIBATES are women who are involved in passionate love affairs. They consider themselves celibate because they are not actually having intercourse, but they come pretty darned close.

TEN COMMANDMENT CELIBATES are committed to abstaining from sex until marriage.

MODERATE CELIBATES remain celibate until they are involved in a monogamous, committed relationship that may or may not lead to marriage.

HEALING CELIBATES deliberately excuse themselves from the dating arena in order to heal from emotional or physical trauma. Some women in this category have suffered domestic violence, rape, or the death of a spouse. Others are recuperating from a physical illness, pregnancy, etc. If they seek medical, spiritual, and/or psychological help, Healing Celibates can go on to enjoy fulfilling sexual relationships. If not, they may become Retired Celibates.

MARRIED CELIBATES. If celibacy is a mutual, conscious choice in a marriage relationship for mutually agreed upon periods of time, it can be a time of growth and healing for both partners. However, too many married people have been forced into celibacy because of illness, mismatched or low sex drives, infidelity, or abuse, which makes it a time of great pain. While the problems inherent in this type of celibacy are beyond the scope of this book, there is no reason why, even in the "driest" of situations, a woman can't maintain her passion for life through the Sensual Celibacy Program.

The way a woman enters into celibacy will determine the quality of her experience initially. For example, if a woman feels "forced" into celibacy because of the traumatic end of a relationship, the absence of sex may feel extremely uncomfortable, and she may desperately seek relief. Or, she may hide within the experience of celibacy so that

CELIBACY WORKS. IT MAKES YOU CLEAR AND FOCUSED. . . . I DON'T THINK CELIBACY IS FOR EVERYBODY FOR THE LENGTH OF TIME THAT I'VE DONE IT. AIDS PROPELLED ME INTO CELIBACY. THE SPIRITUAL AWAKENING CAME LATER.

—JACKEE

she doesn't have to face the world. This is sometimes called "sexual anorexia." The good news is that as a woman completes her mourning, she can begin to practice the sensual form of celibacy this book advocates and allow the healing process to begin. Regardless of how a woman enters into celibacy, there's nothing stopping her from choosing to make the experience a good one.

The above list should not be used to pass judgment or engage in blame or shame. No one type of celibate is better or worse than any other. Each has to contend with its own issues. The list simply represents a variety of reasons and ways women engage in a celibate lifestyle. Nor is the list meant to be all inclusive. There are, theoretically, as many reasons for celibacy and ways of practicing it as there are celibates in the world. The purpose is to help you see where you are in the great scheme of things. The more you can define where you are, the better you will know who you are and how to determine your true agenda for this period, that is, how to accomplish your goals, hopes, and dreams. The more you know, the better equipped you'll be to make the celibacy experience a positive one.

In the past, I considered myself a Moderate Celibate, although I've been a Healing Celibate and have threatened to quit and become a Professional Celibate (i.e., a nun). Now I've resolved to "save myself for my husband."

"But, Donna, you aren't practicing celibacy at all," said Sharon, a married friend of mine, one day as we were eating pizza and minding our children together.

I put down my cheese slice and stared at her in disbelief. Here was a woman, married for fifteen years, getting it and getting it good most nights, and she had the nerve to judge my behavior, decisions, and morality. I was appalled and, I hate to admit, put on the defensive. "I think two and one-half years of not having sex ranks as celibacy," I said furiously.

Sharon adamantly shook her head. "No, what you've been doing is taking breaks in between sexual relationships. That's not celibacy." I was even more furious. All my life I've been judged by family, friends, and society for one "failing" or the other: Donna, you're too sensitive. Donna, you need to go to church. Donna, you need to be a vegetarian. Donna, you need to eat only one meal a day. Donna, you're too heavy, you need to lose weight. Intolerance seems to be the order of the day in America, and now I was being told that I wasn't even not having sex right.

"Celibacy is not doing it until *marriage,*" said Sharon. My dear friend is a married woman with an Old Testament life philosophy, and I knew there was no winning this argument. My life flashed before my eyes, and suddenly I felt sick and tired of people judging me who had never walked in my pumps. I decided to fight back and defend myself as best I could against Sharon's deeply ingrained dogma and her life experiences.

"So," I said, "I should bargain my sexuality for a ring? I have a problem with that."

"All I know is that if you keep doing the same thing over and over again, you're going to get the same results."

She had a point. Yet I couldn't quite make myself believe that premarital sex was the villain preventing me from getting married. Lots of married people I know did it while single, and look at them now. They're married! Sharon did it with her husband before they got married, and look at them now. Married! No, I think that whole *Rules* approach to snatching a man might be good for controlling your own behavior but is way too simplistic to account for all the complexities and dynamics involved in being in a relationship.

"God gave us different laws for good reasons," said Sharon, "although we may not always know what they are. God said, 'Stick to kosher, don't eat shrimp,' and science has discovered that shrimp is high in cholesterol. God said, 'Don't fornicate,' and now we know why. Diseases, unwanted pregnancies—"

"Well," I said, defeated, "I believe in the compassion, love, mercy, and forgiveness part of the Bible." And what I also wanted to say was that my reasons for leaning toward saving sex until after marriage were eminently practical and had little to do with biblical teachings, although I respect them. Premarital sex has not worked for me. Sex attaches me to a man, and when a breakup occurs, I'm too devastated. I no longer choose to go through the emotional roller coaster. I figure, if I postpone sex as long as possible (which can be difficult; after all, I am an earthy woman), then I lessen the risk of pain and suffering if the relationship doesn't work out.

"If you can get the milk for free, why pay for the whole cow?" said Sharon, her last-ditch attempt to convert me to her point of view. Although I didn't appreciate the heifer association, I understood the point. Yet I couldn't shake the feeling of game playing and bargaining: my jewels for his diamond ring.

The conclusion I've come to is this: I've come too far in my quest for self-determination and liberation from social expectations to walk back into a cage of someone else's design. If I decide, after much prayer and soul-searching, to go back to being a Moderate Celibate, then that's my choice. As I lean more toward sex within marriage, however, I trust that God has brought me to the place where God wants me to be.

I hear the cries of teenaged girls and women across the country. "But if I don't have sex with him, he'll leave!" Why should he stay with you when sex is so plentiful and easily available?

There are two answers to that: (1) Because you're an amazingly wonderful, attractive woman and worth the wait. And (2), if he leaves, he was a spoiled little boy throwing a temper tantrum because he couldn't get his own way. He wasn't worth your time after all.

Sex and No Sex

Celibacy is one of the sexiest topics around, because when you talk about celibacy, you're also talking about sex. To feel comfortable in your new role as a woman practicing celibacy, you'll have to come to terms with the sexual side of your being. You're a sexual woman who's not having sex. Just because you've signed a Celibacy Promise doesn't mean that the horniness and the erotic thoughts and memories of hot, steamy nights will go away. They won't. In fact, during the first few months, you'll probably be thinking about sex night and day.

Every woman will bring to her term of celibacy a load of sexual baggage. For some of us, there are few problems, just a healthy, fun-loving attitude about sex. For others, there's a lot of pain associated with sex. Childhood sexual abuse, stranger rape, spousal rape—needless to say, these events traumatically affect how a woman perceives the act. Still others may wonder, What's the big deal?

Wherever you fall in the spectrum, be gentle and kind and forgiving of yourself. Many of us received our education in sex via a book that Mom handed us or a sex education film in health class. At an early age, some of us caught glimpses of pornographic pictures in magazines. Talking openly about sex, the good, the bad, and the weird, is a relatively new phenomenon. As recently as the 1950s, sex was in the closet. Despite all the studies that have been done on sex, we still don't have all the answers. For example, we still don't really know why some women have orgasms and others don't. Although it's used to sell everything from cigarettes to lawn fertilizer, sex is still a mystery in a lot of ways.

The next few questions were designed to provoke you into thinking of your attitudes about sex and how they may need an update. Did your old paradigm serve you? If not, you've got some thinking to do, and now that you're *not* having sex this is the best time to do it. Now you have the distance needed to think clearly about this steamy subject. So get out your trusty journal and get to writing!

First Lessons

+ How old were you when you first learned what really went on during sexual intercourse? What was your reaction? Were you grossed out or did you care one way or the other?

+ What were your early feelings around penises? Your own vagina?

+ Who taught you about sex? Your mother? Friends? Did anyone tell you anything about sex?

+ How was the information transmitted? Verbally, a film, a TV show, a book?

+ Were you taught about contraception?

♦ When was the first time you masturbated? Were you taught or did it just happen? How did you feel about it? What were you taught about it?

Your First Time

Your first experience of sexual intercourse was, no doubt, a landmark time in your life. For better or for worse, it probably continues to affect the quality of your relationships.

♦ How old were you when you had your first sexual experience?

♦ How was it? Was it good or bad?

♦ Did the intercourse hurt?

♦ Where did your first experience occur?

♦ What were you thinking, feeling?

♦ Did you want to get married?

♦ Did you think you were in love?

♦ Did you use contraception? What kind? If not, why?

Your Best Sexual Experience

♦ Describe your best experience. If you haven't had it yet, fantasize.

♦ Do you feel you've had the ultimate sexual experience? What is the ultimate for you?

♦ Would the ultimate be attached to an emotional high, i.e., love? Have you ever had that?

♦ During your best sex, what were you wearing? In your fantasy sex, what would you be wearing?

+ What did your man do to make this the ultimate experience? What did you do?

+ Why was this your best experience?

Your Worst Sexual Experience

+ Describe your worst experience.

+ How old were you?

+ How does this experience affect your sexual relationships today?

+ Why was this experience your worst?

+ Have you ever felt like you've been raped? Have you been raped by a stranger, husband, or date? Have you sought counseling?

+ Have you ever been drugged?

Your Last Sexual Experience

+ Describe your last experience.

+ Who was it with?

+ Is it a good or bad memory? How did it make you feel?

+ Why was it your last experience?

+ Do you think about it a lot?

General Questions

+ Is sex tied up with commitment?

+ Do you like recreational sex?

+ Which do you prefer, committed or not?

+ Is penis size important?

+ Does the image that you have of your body size affect the quality of your sex?

+ Are stimulants a necessary part of your sexual experience?

+ Is your sexual behavior tied into your spiritual beliefs?

+ Do you like phone sex?

+ Do you like your sex tame or are you adventurous?

+ Do you have erotic dreams? What are they like?

+ Is monagamy important to the quality of sex? Why?

+ Do you have to love the men you sleep with? Do you tend to like them?

+ Are you concerned about sexually transmitted diseases?

Again, the purpose of these self-assessment questions is to get you thinking about issues that you might not ordinarily think about. As you explore these questions in your journal, you'll see your sexual paradigm emerge. You may be surprised. There may be contradictions among beliefs, values, and behaviors. Forgive yourself. Be gentle. Our feelings and attitudes about sex are complex. There is beauty, but sex also has its shadow side, which most of us have experienced in one form or another.

Spend as much time as you need on these questions. No doubt, they will jog some memories and ideas. Face them. Do not hide from them. Embrace them, learn from them, and then let them go.

We will emerge from this period of celibacy healthy and whole. Equally important, we will create new sexual paradigms that are more self-empowering. I cannot stress enough, if you need counseling,

Marilyn Monroe and I discussed it often and agreed it would be nice if we could be strong enough in ourselves as women and not just there to make the male audience want to go to bed with us.

—LENA HORNE

get help. Our attitudes about sex are lodged so deeply within our personalities that sometimes it is difficult to unravel them all by ourselves.

But unravel you must if you are to make this journey of self-discovery a meaningful experience. To know oneself is the beginning of unconditional love, and if we are to improve the quality of all of our relationships, including our romantic ones, then we must wipe the sleep from our eyes and wake up to our true selves.

As you're continuing to explore the questions posed in this chapter, remember the solemnity of your Celibacy Promise. If you know nothing else about yourself, know this: that you can be a woman of your word and that you can keep a promise to yourself.

AFFIRMATION: *I am getting to know the real me, and I like what I see. I'm not perfect, but I love myself unconditionally.*

CHAPTER FIVE

Step 3 — Set, Then Pursue, Goals

♦ ♦ ♦

Once you start waking up, there's no going back to sleep. As you learn more and more about yourself—your strengths, weaknesses, hopes, and dreams—you'll see the need to overhaul certain portions of your life. Don't judge or criticize yourself. Just get busy.

A period of celibacy is the perfect moment in your life to engage in strategic life planning. Companies use the process to set their activities on a focused path of growth, and so can you.

If you don't have an agenda for this celibacy period, someone will create one for you. Earthy women without a plan are easy targets for seduction. What are your goals, hopes, wishes, and dreams (1) in your life and (2) for this period of celibacy? Are they man-focused or you-focused? As much as we love them, we've got to take our sights off men. First, let's think of celibacy not as the absence of men or sex but as the fullness of ourselves. This is a radical but absolutely necessary shift in thinking if we are to make this a productive period. Second, let's use this time alone wisely to revisit the key areas in our lives: health (emotional and physical), relationships, education, career, and spirituality. Go back to school, lose weight, start a business, develop a new hobby, learn a new skill, make a career change, commit to a spiritual practice. Here's a good one: Develop male friendships (more on that later). Now is the time to dream big and take risks. The best part of all is that you don't have to compromise with anyone.

Action Planning

Action planning is a process in which you create a map for your life. When corporations engage in strategic planning, the process can take months, even years. If management is truly committed to change, they will allocate a significant portion of resources to planning.

In the last chapters, we laid the foundation for the following exercises. You cannot set goals for your life if you are not in touch with your needs, desires, hopes, and dreams. Keep in mind the information that you gleaned from the previous chapters as you work through the following exercises.

In the mid-90s I helped to facilitate hundreds of strategic-planning workshops with school-community groups throughout the Midwest for the Safe and Drug-Free Schools and Communities Program. You too may have gone through a similar process in your company or community group, but this will probably be the first time you've ever used it to plan for a productive and enjoyable celibacy experience. The steps involved are tried and true, but the application to the Sensual Celibacy Program is brand new.

If you are truly committed to using this period of celibacy to make changes in your life, you will have to allocate a significant amount of time and meditation to completing the activities and worksheets that follow. Take your time as you work through the exercises. If you need to, talk to trusted friends and family members. Tell them what you're up to and that their support is needed. They might help provide perspective on your situation that you lack, or they may just be good listeners.

In the final analysis, trust yourself. You have direct access to all the information and guidance you'll ever need. Just look within. If we ask for help, we will surely receive help. All we have to do is ask, believe, then wait for the answer.

BRAINSTORMING ACTIVITY. I absolutely love doing this exercise and still do it from time to time. Remember all those hopes and dreams you have yet to manifest in your life? Now is the time to let your imagination fly. Give yourself permission to dream and hope again. Set the timer for five minutes and, as quickly as you can, list on a separate sheet of paper all of your hopes, dreams, wishes, and fantasies yet to be realized (and that includes your desire for partnership). No holding back. Let go!

*S*TANFORD UNIVERSITY RESEARCHERS RELEASED A NEW STUDY YESTERDAY WHICH HAS REVEALED A POSITIVE LINK BETWEEN SCIENCE FICTION AND CELIBACY. "FOR SOME REASON," STANFORD'S JANET GEERSON SAID, "WE HAVE FOUND THAT THOSE WHO ENJOY FANTASY-THEMED FILMS, MAGAZINES AND BOOKS, SUCH AS *I, ROBOT* AND *THE HOBBIT,* ARE TWICE AS LIKELY TO ABSTAIN FROM SEX AS THOSE WHO DO NOT."

—*THE ONION* (AN ONLINE HUMOR NEWSPAPER)

ORGANIZE YOUR DREAMS. Wasn't that brainstorming activity a blast? Your list should be pretty long. Take that list of dreams and realistically assess when each dream might be accomplished. Copy the forms below and fill them in on the copy.

IMMEDIATE 0–1 YEAR	SHORT-TERM 1–5 YEARS	LONG-TERM 5+ YEARS

RATE YOUR DREAMS. Now go back to the above list and rank them in order of importance. Rank each period of time separately.

PRIORITIZE YOUR DREAMS. List below the top two dreams for each period. Choose the dreams that you feel most strongly about.

IMMEDIATE 0–1 YEAR	SHORT-TERM 1–5 YEARS	LONG-TERM 5+ YEARS
1.	1.	1.
2.	2.	2.

CONVERT YOUR DREAMS INTO GOAL STATEMENTS. The purpose of these exercises is to help you make the most of your period of celibacy by creating the action plan that will turn your dreams into reality. Converting your dreams into goal statements will help you begin to think about them more concretely. For example, if your dream is to lose weight, your goal statement might read: I want to lose twenty-five pounds in eight months.

IMMEDIATE GOALS

(1) I want to _____.

(2) I want to _____.

SHORT-TERM GOALS

(1) I want to _____.

(2) I want to _____.

LONG-TERM GOALS

(1) I want to _____.

(2) I want to _____.

ACTION PLANS. Planning plus faith plus actions make dreams into reality. On the next three pages you'll find three forms for immediate, short-, and long-term planning. Immediate goals are things you want to work on right away. Short-term goals are accomplishments that you can make happen in six months to two years. Long-term goals might take three to twenty years, or more. This activity is most important in that you will be assigning yourself meaningful action steps with deadlines.

In the first column, list your goal statements from the list above. In column 2, list some action steps that you will need to take to accomplish your goal. For example, if your goal is to lose ten pounds, one of your action steps might be to join a diet club.

In column 3, list the dates you plan to complete the action steps. Give yourself reasonable completion dates and make every effort to meet your deadlines.

In column 4, list the resources that you have at your disposal that will help you get the job done. Back to our weight-loss example: If a nearby park has a great walking path, list it. Resources can also include your own skills, the skills of others, finances, support network, and inner qualities like a strong work ethic, or a kind and generous nature. The resources column is also helpful in seeing what supports are lacking.

Column 5 provides a reality check. It seems to be a law of the universe, but whenever you try to do something positive, life will test your resolve and stamina with some crazy obstacles. Use this column to try and anticipate possible problems and solutions that might arise. Some obstacles might include your own tendency to procrastinate, an unsupportive family member, or the lack of a college degree. While it is important to identify obstacles, it is even more important to plan and move toward overcoming them.

Refer back to your action plans time and again. Fine-tune them if necessary, and by all means, reward yourself as you accomplish each of the action steps. There are few things in life that feel as good as when you achieve your goals. Dare we say, it can be better than sex!

One final thought on action planning: Some of the greatest Professional Celibates the world has ever known, i.e., priests, priestesses, nuns, and monks of all religions, have struggled with the issue of celibacy. Unfortunately, we only hear of Catholic priests, who, unable to stick to their commitment, have used their positions of power to sexually abuse others. No punishment is too harsh for them. But there are others who have come to terms with celibacy and have become some of the greatest lovers of humanity the world has ever known. We might not want to be celibate forever, but we can learn from what we know about the lives of people like the Dalai Lama, Bishop Desmond Tutu, Mahatma Gandhi, and Mother Teresa. Serving others forms a major component of their vocation and helps in great measure to transmute sexual urges into a higher calling. As you continue to refine your strategic plan, I would urge you to consider including an activity that you can do to help make the world a better place. During celibacy so much of our attention is focused inward on our pain, our needs, and our desires that without an outer-directed activity we can lose perspective.

Would you believe? Elvis Presley refused to consummate his relationship with Priscilla until their wedding night.

—FROM JOHN WHITCOMB AND CLAIRE WHITCOMB, GREAT AMERICAN ANECDOTES

Service is a win-win proposition for you and the cause that you choose to give your time to.

IMMEDIATE GOALS	ACTION STEPS	COMPLETION DATES	RESOURCES	OBSTACLES AND WAYS TO OVER-COME THEM
1. I WANT TO:	1.	1.	1.	1.
	2.	2.	2.	2.
	3.	3.	3.	3.
	4.	4.		
	5.	5.		
2. I WANT TO:	1.	1.	1.	1.
	2.	2.	2.	2.
	3.	3.	3.	3.
	4.	4.		
	5.	5.		

SHORT-TERM GOALS	ACTION STEPS	COMPLETION DATES	RESOURCES	OBSTACLES AND WAYS TO OVER-COME THEM
1. I WANT TO:	1.	1.	1.	1.
	2.	2.	2.	2.
	3.	3.	3.	3.
	4.	4.		
	5.	5.		
2. I WANT TO:	1.	1.	1.	1.
	2.	2.	2.	2.
	3.	3.	3.	3.
	4.	4.		
	5.	5.		

LONG-TERM GOALS	ACTION STEPS	COMPLETION DATES	RESOURCES	OBSTACLES AND WAYS TO OVER- COME THEM
1. I WANT TO:	1. 2. 3. 4. 5.	1. 2. 3. 4. 5.	1. 2. 3.	1. 2. 3.
2. I WANT TO:	1. 2. 3. 4. 5.	1. 2. 3. 4. 5.	1. 2. 3.	1. 2. 3.

LIFE-MISSION STATEMENT. Your life-mission statement addresses the questions: What lessons am I supposed to learn? What is my life all about? What is the work that my God would have me do?

Normally you begin the strategic-planning process with a discussion and a brainstorming session around your mission statement. From that statement all goals and action steps flow. I include it at the end of the process for one simple reason: Mission statements can take a long time to conceive—days, months, even years. You may not have that long—you could meet Mr. Wonderful tomorrow! (Now even if you meet him, don't stop this process. A period of celibacy is the ideal time to work on self because you're not so emotionally wrapped up in another person. However, being in a relationship is no excuse for not working to improve your life. The pattern for many women is to get real busy while celibate, but as soon as a man comes along, they lose their minds. No more excuses. Right now, your attitude has got to be that getting yourself together is more important than anything else. It's the one and only priority.)

Work on your life-mission statement, but don't let your ignorance of your purpose prevent you from setting goals and taking steps to make your dreams come true. Hidden in your goals are probably clues to your high calling. As your life mission is revealed to you over time, you'll probably want to revise your goals. Maybe losing weight isn't as important as going back to school. This is not a static process. Try to achieve a balance between flexibility and commitment.

If you know your life mission and have chosen to practice celibacy for a time, this period can be tremendously productive. If you don't know your life mission, there's no better time than the present to do some soul-searching.

Why all this activity? you might ask. Idleness is the great enemy of celibacy. It paves a wide path for all sorts of seductions that you might not yet be ready for. The fact that you are designing your own program based on your own needs, wants, desires, and eventually your life mission ensures that the activities you embark upon will not be just busywork but meaningful and powerful enough to achieve your dreams.

It is the quirkiness of life that just when we are about to make a personal breakthrough in whatever issues have been challenging us, some temptation will come along to test us. In the celibate's case, if she gives in to sex before she is ready, she may find herself having to go back to square one, which is what happened to me. Both of my children were conceived at the threshold of such breakthrough moments—my son on the eve of a career promotion and my daughter as I was beginning to achieve my health and fitness goals. I love my children, but I wish I had had them under different circumstances (marriage) and with *one* man who really loved me. Unfortunately, I allowed loneliness and desperation to creep in both times, and I ended up choosing unwisely. As a result, each time I was forced to start over in a number of ways. Loneliness and temptation are common problems facing passionate women practicing celibacy; however, when a woman has become attuned to her high life calling, she is less at risk for making bad decisions about relationships.

*W*HAT DOES "GOOD IN BED" MEAN TO ME? WHEN I'M SICK AND I STAY HOME FROM SCHOOL PROPPED UP WITH LOTS OF PILLOWS, WATCHING TV, AND MY MOM BRINGS ME SOUP—THAT'S GOOD IN BED.
—BROOKE SHIELDS

In addition to feeling charged about life, you'll attain a clarity of thought. As your life more completely revolves around your mission, you'll want all aspects of your life—from the neighborhood you live in to the friends you keep—to support your work. All sorts of people and situations will continue to flow past you, but you will be blessed with the power of discernment. You'll become increasingly able to distinguish the good from the bad.

This would be a good time to revisit your Celibacy Promise. Are you on track? How do you feel about your promise? Are you having a difficult time keeping it, or has it been smooth sailing? Record your feelings in your journal.

UNDERWEAR EXERCISE. Some changes do not have to take forever, say Maryann V. Troiani and Michael W. Mercer, the authors of a fun book, *Change Your Underwear, Change Your Life.* You can give yourself an emotional lift by simply wearing luxurious underthings.

To peer deeply into the essence of your being, picture underwear you like to wear. Cotton? Silk? High-cut, exposing your entire side and hipbone? Extremely modest, covering every inch possible up to your neck? Or perhaps wearing an itsy-bitsy-teeny . . .

And how about your bra, *if* you are wearing one?

What about the colors? (Troiani and Mercer, p. 220)

Do inventory on your underwear drawer and tell the truth: Do you like what you see? How do those white cotton drawers make you feel? Sexy? I think not! A period of celibacy is precisely the time to feel sexy— not to try and rope in some man but to continue to experience the part of yourself that is all woman. We women are so used to feeling sexual in the context of a relationship that it might be a new and unusual experience to feel this way for you and you alone.

If you can afford to throw those old bloomers away and buy new, sexy ones, then by all means do that. If not, put aside money to splurge on one sexy lingerie ensemble. If you make a frivolous purchase, make it this one!

AFFIRMATION: *I refuse to let myself go just because I don't have a man. I am a sexy, sensuous, attractive woman inside and out!*

CHAPTER SIX

Step 4— Heal Your Soul

I've never felt this kind of pain. It leaves you raw and vulnerable. Now when you're faced with something that painful, you have two choices. You can do down, go under—just cave in out of the fear of what it means to be single again. Or you can say this is to open a door that I've never even thought of opening.

—Jane Fonda

There's nothing quite like the pain that follows the breakup of a relationship or the death of a spouse. Nowhere to run, nowhere to hide. In *Care of the Soul,* Thomas Moore says that achieving inner healing requires an "interplay of spirituality and soul. . . . A spiritual life of some kind is absolutely necessary for psychological 'health.'"

My second big celibacy event occurred when I became pregnant with my first child. The father walked out on me in my fourth month, and there I was, stuck, lonely, and alone. I was growing as big as a house, with no ring on my finger. Everywhere I turned, I saw married couples pushing baby buggies. If it wasn't for the unconditional love and support I received from my family, I don't know how I would have made it through that nightmare.

I was in serious denial about my predicament. I wasn't *that* kind of woman. I had not been raised to be a single parent. I was ashamed of myself. I was blessed with a beautiful baby boy, but with that blessing came an emotional depression I had not seen the likes of since my divorce. There were times when I literally could not breathe. It was an ongoing soap opera, but I thank my God for healing. It does come.

Shortly after the abandonment, I reclaimed the faith of my girlhood. Late one night in September 1985, I lay down on my living room floor and reclaimed my Christian faith. It was the end of the line for me, and I knew it. So I did what so many millions of women and men have done since the beginning of time—I surrendered my life to a Higher Power, admitted that I was incompetent in handling my affairs, and asked for guidance and healing. As I lay on the floor not really expecting an answer, yet daring to hope for one, I began to have the strangest sensation of garbage—balls of crumpled paper, rusty nails—rising up and out of my body. That was sign enough for me. I believed I had been heard.

> THE REAL SECRET
> OF [ROOSEVELT'S] SEX
> LIFE WAS, PROBABLY,
> THAT THERE WAS NO
> SEX LIFE . . .
>
> —GARY WILLS

Most important, I needed to know that although I felt alone at the moment, the most awesome Presence in the universe loved me. My God seemed closer to me than my own breath, and this was the healing balm I needed. I still had four more months of pregnancy to endure, and then the real work of raising a child by myself would begin. In all honesty I can't say that my life got any easier. But I can say that for the first time since I had become involved with men, I felt truly loved and wanted.

My worst trial led to my greatest spiritual blessing. I revisited Christianity by watching televangelists and going to a Pentecostal church—but I soon gave all that up. I stopped listening to the beliefs and dogma of others and began to try and hear Spirit for myself. As a result, I shed some old beliefs and acquired some new ones. I deprogrammed myself from my old conditioning and fear of God, and began to acquaint myself with the God of love, mercy, and compassion.

Because Christianity has shaped so much of our views on celibacy, even those of us in the secular world, it is important to reiterate that celibacy is not just for Christians—or Muslims, Jews, or Buddhists, for that matter. No organization owns it. Celibacy is available to anyone, regardless of race, gender, sexual orientation, religion, or views on premarital sex.

Ironically, in all the many years I spent in the church, I heard a lot of hellfire and damnation preaching against premarital sex, but not once did I hear from the ministers or the learned church women how to make that happen, at least not in a way that made sense to me. Singles workshops are often led by married people, and they focus on preparing the participants for marriage. The institution that so loudly proclaims the "no fornication" rule turns a deaf ear to the physical, spiritual, and psychological needs of its single members. Some progressive churches do pay attention, but from what many women and men in the church have told me, the neglect tends to be systemwide.

I wish I could say that once I left the church, my life made a turn for the better. Actually, for a moment, it did. During my first pregnancy, I gained a lot of weight, so I put myself on a health and fitness program to lose weight and firm up. I began to look and feel better than I had in a long time. Unfortunately, because I had neglected my soul wounds, history was destined to repeat itself. Seven years after meeting Father #1, I met Father #2. Seven years after becoming pregnant with my son, I became pregnant with my daughter—almost to the same day. In fact, both of my children have birthdays in February. Father #1 walked out on me in August. Father #2 walked out on me in August. During pregnancy #1, I gained forty pounds. I gained forty more during pregnancy #2.

However, there were also some key differences in the circumstances. During pregnancy #1, I thought I was going to die from grief. During pregnancy #2, I wanted to *kick ass*—the father's, that is. I was furious. I wanted to burn this man's house down. I wanted to do him bodily harm. (Needless to say, I was in the anger stage of dying.)

Strangely, my anger energized me and made me attractive to men. I hadn't had so much male attention since high school. I went out on dates and made it a point to look cute at all times. I also discovered a therapeutic technique that I would heartily recommend to all women suffering heartbreak: laughter. Watch funny shows and listen to comedy tapes. Norman Cousins healed himself of an illness by watching tapes of old comedy show reruns, and I survived my nine months of pregnancy by listening to Eddie Murphy and Sinbad.

I don't excuse what these men did, but when history repeats itself so blatantly, you're getting a wake-up call. You have to do some honest soul-searching. You have to examine your behavior, values, issues, up-bringing—everything. So I did. I went through the hard heart work with the help of my sisters and a couple of close friends and made some breakthroughs. I worked on the old, destructive relationship patterns from childhood. I never wanted to repeat this history again.

Heart work can be grueling, but the benefits are well worth the effort. I wish I could paint you a pretty picture, but I can't. You have to confess and own your issues, and that's not always fun. Yes, those men treated me badly, and what goes around comes around. But I invited them into my life, and I had to own up to that. I made myself a victim. I had sex with them before I knew enough about them to make an intelligent decision.

All kinds of people, good and bad, will parade through your life, but your state of mind and your emotional health will determine to whom you'll be attracted and pay attention. (Like attracts like.) During Celibacy Periods 1 through 4, I doubt that I would have met the types of men that I am proud to call my friends today. Men have come and gone, but today, I'm happy to say, the good ones seem to be staying. That says a lot about how much I've healed. I used to be easily charmed by bad boys, but today I see them for the insecure, emotionally wounded souls that they are. Most important, I now understand how my old programming conspired to make me attractive to these guys.

I went after my healing with a vengeance because I never wanted to go through such pain ever again. I wanted my healing more than money, more than a man.

That's how badly you've got to want to heal from grief, bad relationships, and bad periods of celibacy. If you don't take your healing into your own hands, you're bound to repeat history until you get it right. It's a law of the universe.

Just ask yourself one question: Do you really want to go through all that again? Is being with a man, any old man, worth all the pain and agony that comes with relationships made from desperate choices? When you keep doing the same things, you're going to keep getting the same results.

Never before have so many self-help books been printed, tapes produced, and workshops organized. Women can go to spiritual leaders and psychologists of every stripe and persuasion. Help is out there, if only we'd grab our healing like the lifeline that it is. Some of us still feel it is a weakness to seek help when we're hurting, but it's not. It's a supreme act of courage.

HOWARD [STERN] STARTED REFERRING TO ME AS A "BLACK WIDOW" WHO TRAVELED TO EXOTIC PLACES TO SUCK THE LIFE OUT OF YOUNG MEN. HIS REASONING WENT THAT MY SEXUALITY SEEMED TO SURFACE FOR A TIME, THEN DISAPPEAR. . . . LIKE SPOCK, THE VULCAN CHARACTER FROM *STAR TREK,* I HAD A MATING SEASON EVERY FEW YEARS. THE TRUTH OF IT WAS THAT I STILL DIDN'T FEEL WORTHY OF LOVE AND WAS AFRAID TO FEEL ANYTHING TOO DEEPLY.

—ROBIN QUIVERS

Sex and Your Soul

When the soul is neglected, it doesn't just go away; it appears symptomatically in obsessions, addictions, violence, and loss of meaning.

—Thomas Moore, *Care of the Soul*

You can't touch the soul or measure its weight on a scale. But when your soul is in crisis, you know it because it makes itself heard, loudly and clearly. You know your soul is screaming for attention when

+ At work, time moves at a snail's pace. You're forever watching a clock that never moves.

+ Arguments with a partner feel like an old show in syndication—same old tired reruns, nothing new.

+ The pastimes that used to give you so much pleasure are now boring and meaningless.

+ All your needs, and some of your wants, are being met, but still you feel depressed and deprived.

+ You have an irresistible urge to indulge in taboo or even dangerous activities.

+ The material world no longer holds any fascination for you. You long for a mystical experience.

Remember the story that grabbed the nation's attention—the mass suicide of thirty-eight Heaven's Gate members? A LIFE OF CELIBACY, ISOLATION screamed the *Chicago Sun-Times* headline, and my first thought was, oh, no, now they're linking celibacy with dementia. How will we healthy sensual celibates ever live this one down? Not only were the members celibate, the males had been surgically castrated. My second thought was, they didn't trust themselves to keep their commitment to abstain from sex, so the best solution they could think of was to cut off their balls. "Why not end the battle with the sex drive?" reasoned Dick Joslyn, a former member who had been with the cult for fifteen years.

Clearly the souls of the Heaven's Gate members were in crisis, and they attempted to alleviate their malaise through spiritual seeking that was excessive, ungrounded, and did not include soul work. They sought to fill their lives with meaning, but made the fatal mistake of handing over control of their souls to Marshall Applewhite, their leader. The members submitted to martial law that controlled their lives from the time they woke up in the morning until the time they went to bed. Even their time of death was decided for them. Instead of receiving the meaning that their souls craved, they gave up personal responsibility, and with it, their freedom.

The Heaven's Gate case is extreme, but I mention it here because it poignantly depicts what desperate people are capable of doing when their souls are in crisis. I trust that you will not go so far as to take your own life, but if you are experiencing a crisis of the soul, you must ask yourself some hard questions. Have you handed over your power to another person? Freedom requires responsibility. Is it easier for you to just go with the flow of someone else's design? When you give up responsibility for your life, you're neglecting the needs of your soul.

You may blame your problems on the lack of a man in your life, but consider this: Your problems may have little to do with your single state and everything to do with your neglect of your own soul. Many of the feelings you experience when alone you probably felt when you were last with a man. The difference was you didn't have to pay attention to your unease while a man was in your space. But now that you're alone, all the you-know-what is hitting the fan. You can try to run away—that's what rebounding is all about—but eventually, your issues will catch up with you. If not now, then later. It's a law of the universe.

We've talked a lot about the agonies that often accompany a term of celibacy, but equally important to the celibate are the issues that continue to arise in relationships, especially during sexual intercourse. One of the best times to self-analyze is when you're having sex, because it is then that all your symptoms come to the surface—especially if you barely know the man. But who wants to self-analyze during sex? All we want to do is feel, we don't want to think. Uncomfortable feelings may nag at us, but we silence them by focusing on the other person.

Lots of us are having sex with men before we're ready. Think back to those times. Why did you do it? What part of yourself did you have to silence? Without a doubt, some part of your soul had to shut down so that you could go on automatic.

More Sex Questions

Sex often occurs within an emotional haze of fear, anxiety, doubt, and guilt, not love. The next series of questions is designed to get you thinking about the impact of your sexual behavior on your emotional health. You should begin to see where the healing work needs to concentrate.

These suggestions should not suggest a condemnation of sex! Far from it. I want us all to have better, hotter sex when that day comes. But first, you have to heal from old wounds and self-destructive programming around men, relationships, and sex. So get out your journal and start writing.

+ Many of us who were raised in the church still have lingering guilt when we have premarital sex. Childhood conditioning is a merciless taskmaster. Sometimes we never entirely shed the residue effects, even after therapy and decades of experience. Are guilt and sex linked in your mind? If so, does it affect the quality of your sex? Your celibacy?

+ Are fear and sex linked in your mind? Are you terrified of getting pregnant or catching a disease? How enjoyable have past sexual experiences been with this mind-set?

+ What happens to your soul when you have sex with a man you fear is repulsed by your body because of plumpness or perceived less-than-ideal body parts? What happens to your soul when you try and hide your body by turning off the lights or wearing clothes to bed?

+ What happens to your soul when you have sex with a man you fear will leave you? What happens to your soul when you try and use sex to keep him? What happens when he leaves after he's had sex with you?

+ Have your sexual experiences been tainted with even the slightest hint of fear, discomfort, anxiety, or shame? Usually

these feelings operate just below the threshold of consciousness, and we keep them at bay by focusing on our partner.

✦ Can you remember a time when you had sex freely and without reservation? Nobody pressured you or tried to make you
feel guilty. Sex was entirely your idea and it felt good. When
your term of celibacy ends and you're ready to have sex again,
this should be your state of mind all the time! Use this time
alone to resolve these issues—and do it for yourself Yes, the
more emotionally healthy you are, the better your sex should
be, although great sex is not the goal of the Sensual Celibacy
Program (it's a nice side benefit). The goal is your well-being
and happiness.

If you've been working the Sensual Celibacy Program thus far,
you've made a promise to vacation from sex for at least six months, and
you've set some goals and seriously considered your life mission. You
should be proud of what you've done so far.

Still, there are probably some issues that nag you and pull on your
heartstrings. Bedtime is probably the loneliest time of day for singles,
and it's then when all the old issues scream for attention.

The good news is that the pain doesn't have to last forever. Healing
is available to you, if you go after it with all the enthusiasm and clever-
ness you use to snare Man. The other day I was talking to a man about
celibacy, and he said that he hoped I would include religion in the book.
By now, I hope I've made my position clear: No religion "owns" celibacy.
(Nor do I think Jesus, Mary, Muhammad, or the Buddha are owned by
the religions that claim them, but that's an argument for another book.)
However, celibacy should be infused with the deep spirituality, not the
facade, of the religion you may claim. I can't imagine how an atheist
would survive the long dark nights of the soul that most celibates face,
but as long as she turns inward, she too can draw on powerful inner resources.

The following are ways that you can begin to integrate your celibacy
practice with soul and spirituality.

CULTIVATE A SENSE OF THE SACRED. In twelve-step programs, recovering addicts are encouraged to seek out a Higher Power in order to begin the healing process. Organized religions worship specific deities. In the New Age movement believers meditate on and seek the guidance of the High Self. Even women who profess no religion or transcendent beliefs have a sense of the sacred in their lives when they're tending their gardens, watching children play, or advocating for a righteous cause.

Whatever our approach to spirituality, whatever our professed beliefs, it is human nature to revere and seek out the sacred. It's all about our lives having meaning. We need to know that we're not just taking up empty space in the universe. There is a purpose to our existence on planet earth, and it is sacred.

PRAY. Church teachings tell women to abstain from sex until marriage, and I have known some women who have stayed faithful for years. Their passion for God keeps their course steadfast. The passionate response of celibate women to the touch of the Holy Spirit suggests that deep down, these are some very earthy women whose sexuality, at least during church service, has been transmuted through praise and worship. For most of them, the ideal is marriage, so I often wonder how they feel about not expressing the sexual side of themselves. Don't they feel like they're missing out?

Not necessarily. In a way, Protestant celibate women remind me of Catholic nuns who relate to Jesus in an intensely intimate way. Both groups speak of this sacred relationship to Jesus as a marriage. Some of us may have difficulty relating to this concept, but keep an open mind. If not a Divine Spouse, how about a Divine Friend? For a woman practicing celibacy, a form of spousal prayer can heal her sense of unworthiness and the feeling of not being loved, for in this type of prayer she receives *unconditional love.* God the Creator of all the universe is so huge that it can be difficult to wrap our thoughts and emotions around God. Through daily dialogues with your Divine Friend, you'll feel the love, compassion, mercy, and forgiveness you'll need to begin the healing process.

How to begin this most intimate of spiritual relationships? I have a friend who simply went out into the woods one day and asked her Beloved to marry her. She says they both recited vows and never did a woman feel more loved. Some time later she met and married a man, but she always remembered her spiritual wedding day as the most special event of her life.

*A*BSTINENCE MAKES THE HEART GROW FONDER.

—KNOX BURGER

If you'd like to engage in this intensely intimate form of prayer, I offer you the following guided visualization. Sit back, close your eyes, and relax. Play soft music or burn incense—whatever helps you attain a state of reverence. I prefer silence.

Breathe deeply to enter a state of profound relaxation. When you feel calm, ask your God to infuse you and embrace you with blessings and protective healing light. Know that you are in God's loving arms and no harm will come to you. You are safe.

Seek a mental picture of your Friend. Maybe it's a holy angel, an avatar, or the Messiah who once walked the earth. See the face and body clearly. The clothes. Note the facial features, the color of the skin. Hear the voice, feel the skin, stroke the hair.

Now feel love and warmth emanating from your Friend. See your Friend take your hands. Hear your Friend say, "I love you. Everything's going to be all right. I'm here for you. You'll never be alone."

Take a moment and bask in the warm, radiant sunshine of unconditional love. It feels so good to be loved like this.

Now ask your Friend for the best place to meet. You can meet anywhere in heaven or on earth. This will be your secret place. Whenever you need companionship, go there and know that you will never be alone. Take some time to get used to this place. Enjoy the companionship of your Friend. Stay as long as you like.

Now, before you open your eyes, thank your Friend for the love and companionship. Ask if there are any parting words. Wait a few moments. Even if you don't hear anything, give thanks for this gift and know that answers to all questions will be forthcoming.

DEVELOP A SPIRITUAL PRACTICE. Every day you need to do something that reminds you of your divine connection and feeds your soul. I would strongly recommend a practice that has a physical component to ground it with sensuality. Here are some suggestions:

✦ Yoga—great for keeping the body limber, toned, and strong, and the mind focused

✦ Qi chung—promotes physical strength and health, and develops an awareness of energy fields that flow through and around the body

✦ Muslim prayer—devout Muslims pray five times per day, facing the east, and they pray with their entire bodies. As you pray, kneel, stretch your arms high above your head, then lower your torso and arms down to the ground.

✦ Sufi prayer—the whirling dervishes spin so fast I get dizzy just watching them, but I hear that the spinning activates the seven chakra energy bodies and excites mystical states. (Watch children. They spin all the time, and they're always spaced out!)

✦ Christian praise and worship—lots of dancing and singing simple, sweet, loving lyrics. Lots of fun, inspires awe and reverence for the Divine.

To engage even more of your senses, burn incense and play inspirational, motivational music.

EXPERIENCE NATURE. Our souls need beauty, love, spirituality, and purpose. We behave irrationally, not because we're crazy or evil sinners, but because we're trying to get our soul needs met. The problem is, we look for beauty, love, spirituality, and purpose in all the wrong places. We lack the skills and knowledge to take care of our souls.

And is it any wonder? Ours is not the most soulful culture on the planet. Far from it. The traditional avenues of soul care—art, literature, dance, music, nature, meaningful work, religion—are little more than industries to be factored into the GNP.

Ask your soul, Soul, how does your garden grow? Is the soil of your soul dry or fertile? Are there flowers or weeds?

I tend my soul's garden with frequent trips to nature, which in Chicago means the Forest Preserves. Lake Michigan satisfies my need for massive quantities of water. If only we had mountains, my life would be complete.

I wish that the Hale-Bopp comet had not become associated with so much pain and death. I had the great fortune to see it with my own two eyes during a trip to California. Late one night my cousin Gino drove me to the top of the mountain city of Rancho Palos Verdes, and there it was, switching its tail, flirting with all the other celestial bodies.

For so long I defined myself by the man in my life. . . . For the first time in my life I'm not afraid to be alone— and I'm loving every minute of it.

—CHER

When seeing something like that and understanding some of the science behind it, there's no way you can feel lonely or depressed. I mean, the comet was zooming a zillion miles per hour, but it looked like it was standing still. Awesome!

BE GRATEFUL. We talked about gratitude in chapter 1, but we discuss it again here because it is a prerequisite to inner soul healing. There have been times when I was in such pain, all I could manage was, "Thank you, God, for my life." Prayers of gratitude help you focus on the blessings, rather than lack, in your life.

FORGIVE. One of the biggest obstacles to healing that celibate women must contend with are the grudges that they hold against ex-boyfriends and ex-spouses. If other women were involved, them too. And yes, you have to forgive all of them.

Look, the forgiveness is not so much for them, but for you. Think of the person causing you the most pain right now. Okay, now feel that emotion in your body. Where is it? Your stomach? Your heart? Your chest? Every time you feel rage in that body part, poisons are congregating there. The longer you keep forgiveness at bay, the greater your risk of illness. I know how difficult it is to give up anger, but you have to do it. I have to do it. Let's do it together: Pray with me:

I need help with forgiveness. I can't forgive, but I know that I need to. I'm angry and I hurt. For my own sake, I will work on letting the bad feelings go. It's more important for me to go on with my life than for me to stay mad. I will forgive and let go. And So It Is.

LOVE YOURSELF UNCONDITIONALLY. Low self-esteem is like the weather. We all talk about it, but we don't do anything about it. We've all heard this bit of wisdom, but it bears repeating: You won't be able to love anyone well if you don't love yourself first. There's nothing like a healthy dose of unconditional self-love to heal a broken heart and stimulate a sense of the sacred in your life. All the great spiritual traditions talk about the healing power of unconditional love. That means you love yourself without reservation—despite all your failures and weaknesses. Read the following great words aloud. This is a love song to yourself:

> *Love is patient,*
> *love is kind.*
> *It does not envy,*
> *it does not boast,*
> *it is not proud.*
> *It is not rude, it is not self-seeking,*
> *it is not easily angered,*
> *it keeps no record of wrongs.*
> *Love does not delight in evil*
> *but rejoices with the truth.*
> *It always protects, always trusts,*
> *always hopes, always perseveres.*
> *Love never fails.*
> —1 CORINTHIANS 14:6
> *(New International Version)*

LOVE PASSIONATELY. A few years ago, a book about women loving too much was published. How can you put a limit on your soul's capacity to experience that feeling we call love? Love in action, that's a different story. We don't have to be stupid. Love with all your heart, but behave wisely. Just because you love a man doesn't mean that you have to be with him. Trying to suppress love because a relationship isn't meant to be is to deny a need of the soul. Allowing yourself to feel love, despite the situation, is a liberating process. Whether or not your love is reciprocated is beside the point. Your emotional well-being is the point.

Also, there's more to love than romance. Love your children, your family, your friends, your coworkers. Love your pets. Love a cause so much that you volunteer your time to it. Love your work so much that you give it your best.

RECONSTRUCT YOUR FAMILY STORY. Family trees, of course, document the names and birth and death dates, as well as extended family branches. Your family's story is not so much concerned with exact dates, but more with the key situations (male-female relationships, careers, child rearing, etc.) that informed the lives of your immediate and extended family members, past and present. While we assume personal responsibility for the decisions we make and the course of our lives, the values, behaviors, and attitudes that were handed down to us have made their mark, whether consciously or unconsciously, on how we handle our affairs. We learn about ourselves when we study the lives of those who came before us. Many of our inner crises have ancestral, even ethnic and racial origins. It takes determination and a supreme act of will to neutralize the effects of the family curse on your life.

In this exercise, you'll use the family tree to tell your family's story. As far back as you can, get names, dates (approximates are okay), and kinship ties. Draw it or describe it in narrative, either way. Unless you want to, you don't have to get county records and that kind of thing. County records would not tell you the loves and sorrows of your ancestors anyway, and that's what you want to know. The best approach is to interview other family members and go treasure hunting for letters and artifacts in attics, basements, and so on.

Once you get a picture of the lives of your relatives, try to come up with what you perceive to be the themes of their lives. If you remember from your high school English class, a theme statement briefly summarizes what the entire story is about. For example, in Great-aunt Ruth's story you might write something like: "Married Great-uncle Ed in 1905.

She wanted to be a singer, but had twenty-five children instead. Stoic, efficient, never smiled. He was stern and undemonstrative. They never seemed to talk to each other."

This soul work will provide information about the behaviors, motivations, intentions, conditioning, and values that have been passed down to you through teaching and osmosis. In particular, you'll want to find out how the female members of your family conducted their love relationships. Also, what were their passions—what kinds of hobbies, activities, etc., did they love to do? Any secret longings? I'd suggest you do this activity during the natural times of the year when your family gets together—family reunions, holidays, weddings, deaths, births of babies, etc. Most important, don't look upon this exercise as work. The sleuthing should be fun and very enlightening.

DICK CAVETT ONCE ASKED BETTE DAVIS WHEN SHE STOPPED BEING A VIRGIN. SHE COUNTED TO TEN AND DECIDED TO ANSWER HIM. "I SAID, 'WHEN I MARRIED MY FIRST HUSBAND.' THEN, AFTER A LONG SILENCE, I SAID, 'AND IT WAS HELL WAITING.'"

—FROM JOHN WHITCOMB AND CLAIRE WHITCOMB, *GREAT AMERICAN ANECDOTES*

About a year before my paternal grandmother died, my sisters and I had long conversations with her about her life. A widow, she had raised her two boys by herself, and so I shouldn't have been surprised when one day, after patiently listening to me whine about not having a husband, she asked me, "What do you need a husband for? You can do okay by yourself." She was the first person to suggest to me that my celibate, single state did not need fixing, and at the time, it was a novel and shocking idea. I must have paled when she said it because she quickly came back with, "Well, I guess you're young yet." No, Grandma, I'm not ready to give up on men just yet. Still, her comment helped me to see how, just like her, I was raising my son (my daughter hadn't been born yet) by myself and I wasn't doing too badly. Just like her, I had found strength within myself to do what I had to do. I didn't crumble and die. As painful as my life had been, I was still carrying on, just like she did.

This exercise will help you understand the strengths and curses that have been passed down to you in ways that you might now understand only barely. The information you'll uncover will provide significant pieces of the mystery that is you.

TALK TO A SOUL DOCTOR. During times of soul crisis, the soul has a need to talk things out. Talking to friends is great, but you'll also need the objectivity of someone who is trained to counsel. One great way to make a connection is to attend some of the many consciousness-raising workshops that are given all across the country. Another way is to ask friends and family members for recommendations. The best way is to trust inner guidance to lead you to the right person. When the patient is ready, the doctor will appear.

CRY. There are times when I cry so hard, it feels like I am crying for the entire world. Afterward, the grief lifts and I feel like the air after a summer rain—cleansed and refreshed. Crying is good for the soul and your physical health. It releases tension that would otherwise stay bottled up inside your body.

LAUGH.
Friend 1: Girl, I got me some last night.
Friend 2: Oh, yeah? Was it good? Did you love it?
Friend 1: Yeah, girl, best sleep I've had in years.
When was the last time you had a good laugh, the kind that erupts from your belly and brings tears to your eyes? Because I have a tendency to take everything way too seriously, I go after laughter with a vengeance. I love going to comedy clubs and watching funny movies. I watch cartoons with my children. And I love a good dirty joke—the raunchier, the better. (I don't question my soul, I just feed it as best I can!)

EXERCISE. Block out fifteen minutes today for a walking (or jogging) meditation in nature. Dress comfortably and find a safe, beautiful place to walk and meditate. Start out by walking at an easy pace. Once you've established a comfortable rhythm, say (to yourself) one of the following phrases:

+ I am a beautiful, intelligent woman.

+ Divine energy flows through me now.

+ I forgive myself. I forgive _____.

+ I'm a beautiful, sexy woman.

+ I love myself unconditionally.

+ I am healed.

+ I am lovable.

'D GONE THROUGH AN ENTIRE YEAR OF CELIBACY BASED ON MY FEELING THAT LUST WAS THE DIRECT CAUSE OF BIRTH WHICH WAS THE DIRECT CAUSE OF SUFFERING AND DEATH . . .

—RECORDING ARTIST MORRISSEY

Or come up with your own affirmation based on your goals and life mission. Say the affirmation in rhythm with your walking. The goal is to be mindful of each step and the sentiment of the affirmation. When you really get good at this, coordinate your breathing with the rhythm you've established. If your thoughts stray, that's okay. Just gently come back to your affirmation.

How have you been doing on your Celibacy Promise? Have you kept your promise to yourself? Sometimes inner healing can be more painful than the incident we're healing from, but don't give up, and don't give in to temptation. In the next chapter, you'll learn some fun ways to strengthen your celibacy practice.

AFFIRMATION: *Today I stop to listen to what my soul is trying to tell me. I will heed the needs of my soul. I am healing my soul.*

CHAPTER SEVEN

Step 5—
Strengthen Your
Celibacy Practice

I've decided that a period of celibacy is in order for me now. . . . I chart my menstrual cycles and notice that I feel increased sexual desire at ovulation. I am free now to feel it but not to act on it. It is simply part of how I am reclaiming my own body's sensual wisdom.

—Christiane Northrup, M.D., "Karen," Women's Bodies, Women's Wisdom: Creating Physical and Emotional Health and Healing

Loneliness and horniness are two of the biggest obstacles to a successful celibacy practice. Many women have thrown in the towel rather than endure one more cold night in a manless bed. Otherwise strong women who have taken the corporate world by storm wither at the sight of their empty beds.

The empty bed is about more than the absence of sex. The empty bed represents the lack of a love relationship and all that involves—companionship, sharing, soul mate stuff. Even after a few months of celibacy and the hormones have finally calmed down, the emotional memories of love remain. Too often, we let the empty bed catapult us out into the night, looking for love in all the wrong ways and in all the wrong places. If you don't get a grip at the beginning of your practice, you run the risk of breaking your promise to yourself, and as a woman of your word, you wouldn't want to do that.

So far, we've talked quite a bit about inner healing and self-discovery. Many abstaining women are confused and in pain about their celibate state, so it was necessary to deal with the heart and identity issues first. If you've been doing the exercises, especially writing (or taping) in your journal most days, you should start gaining insights about yourself. Maybe you're even beginning to feel better about not having a man in your life right now. Maybe you're starting to heal from old wounds. Maybe you're beginning to see the wisdom of taking a vacation from sex if you're not in a monogamous, committed, loving, healthy relationship. That's great! Feel proud of your progress and reward yourself generously with pats on the back and some self-beautification, like a manicure or new hairstyle.

Although everything written thus far was designed to help you strengthen your celibacy practice, this chapter provides some specific strategies to get some platonic fun into your life and to manage your raging hormones (you earthy woman!).

Play

I love to watch my children play. They're so good at it. They run, skip, and jump with such joy and Zen-like mindfulness that I envy them. Watching children at play is like watching little Buddhas meditate. They are totally in the present and only the Muzak of the ice cream truck has the power to distract them.

My own ability to play disintegrated when I discovered boys. The rush I used to feel when swinging, roller-skating, jumping rope, and riding my bicycle was replaced by liking a boy, longing for a boy, hoping the boy liked me back, desperately hoping the boy would call. I gave up my toys the moment boys entered the picture.

Interestingly, boys never gave up their toys or games for me—or any other girls. Boys may grow into manhood, but they never lose their ability to play. Even middle-aged men go through a "second childhood." The pursuit and capture of women is just one game among many. Men are so good at playing that they can transform the most dreary task into a party. I love Tim "the tool man" on *Home Improvement*. He makes washing clothes or baking a gingerbread house an adventure. His tools are his toys, and he never passes up an opportunity to jack up some lowly household appliance with more horsepower, to the dismay of his killjoy, nonplaying wife.

The writer of *Toy Story* really understood the mind of boys at play. A male friend of mine says that when boys play with toys, they infuse their inner being into them. They are not just pretending; the game is real. The toys really do come alive. At first I thought my friend was exaggerating, but I have to admit, watching my son at play more closely has given me a new perspective—and a profound respect for the ability of the male species to play. At twelve years old, an age I used to think was much too old for toys, my son is still playing with action figures, dreaming up scenarios, rigging up contraptions with rubber bands, string, and other junk so that his men can fly, bungee jump, conquer, and rule.

Men know how to play. They play basketball and tag football, watch TV, raid corporations, fiddle with gadgets, and I have yet to meet a man who does not love playing video games. I believe that one of the most important functions of men in marriage is to play with the kids, boys and girls. Single mothers, if there is no man around, find one (hire one) to play with your kids.

I have never known a man to give up his Sunday morning basketball game for me. I don't care how good the loving was on Saturday night, he's packing his duffle bag on Sunday morning. Which, I'm ashamed to say, has, on more than one occasion, left me with absolutely nothing to do except sit by the phone and wait for his call. Over the years I've made that classic mistake so many women make: Since sex was my only play activity, I was totally dependent on men to have fun. The rest of my life was consumed with work. When I gave up the games and toys that gave me pleasure, I screwed myself. I even gave up dancing for my ex-husband! I had nothing left in my life but work, work, and more work. Exercise was work. Making money was work. Going to church was work. Getting beautified at the hair salon was work. Apart from sex, even relationships were work!

We women have given up the joy of running, climbing, and jumping for sex. By doing so, we're ignoring a huge realm of experience that can give us the endorphin rush we need and crave at times. All work and no play makes for a very dull celibacy practice. Some of our childhood enthusiasm for play could be recaptured during exercise, but even then we're "working out." As long as we're in a relationship, we can play at sex, so we come to depend on our playmates for good times and good feelings. But what if there's no man around to give us that special feeling? Does it mean that we have to deny ourselves? Do we have to endure celibacy with grim determination? Does celibacy have to be another day at the office?

According to classical mythology, because Pygmalion was disgusted by the women of Cyprus and was without a wife, he swore himself to celibacy.

Hell, no! One day, while at the park with my children, I asked myself the question, Why should these kids have all the fun? I walked over to the swing stations and stared for a long time. There were many kids around, and I didn't want to embarrass myself or my children, but there was this one swing that was calling my name. It was still and empty and inviting. I remembered the rush I used to feel as a girl when my father used to push me—the sweep of wind across my face, the brush of leaves against my shoes if I stretched my legs long enough, the rush toward the ground, the lift into the sky. I just had to get on that swing!

So I did. I squeezed my ample behind into a swing designed for a child's small one, ran my feet along the sand, and pushed off. I didn't go very high, but oh, what a relief. The sensation was heavenly, just as I remembered. I think we adults should start a new swingers movement. You can have all the playmates you want. It's not about sex, but flying high.

Dolls and female action figures came back into my life a couple of years after I began my first conscious celibacy practice. It was a productive time, but I often worked much too hard, and sometimes my life was much too serious. Dolls opened up my eyes to the vastness of the play spectrum in which sex and romance form just one band. No, I don't get an erotic rush from my dolls, but I do feel happy when I play with them. That's money in the bank for me.

My dolls speak foreign languages and represent many exotic cultures. They are fairies, mermaids, superheroes, angels, and queens. They are brides and glamour women. My dolls dance! My dolls resonate with some deeply hidden aspects of myself that have been yearning to break free for many years now. These dolls represent the wild woman aspect of my nature that my middle-class, conservative upbringing blocked from coming forth.

Doll collecting can be expensive for women on a budget, but action figures are relatively cheap. Action figures aren't just for boys anymore; they're for girls too (and women who are rediscovering the joys of play). Batgirl, She-Hulk, Storm (X-Men), and the Goddess (Spawn). The bad girls are cool too: Catwoman and Poison Ivy (Batman), Bride of Venom (Spiderman), and Lady Deathstrike (X-Men). These action figures are three-dimensional representations of comic book characters. They have superhuman strengths and powers. Given all the work we do in a day, they are toys women can relate to.

Now, we've been around the block a few times. It may be difficult to make the shift from craving romance to playing with dolls, but keep an open mind. It can be done. Just because you're celibate right now doesn't mean that you have to give up sensuality and fun. You're just shifting your attention from one narrow (though terribly exciting) band to the huge, adventure-filled territory of the play spectrum. The "inner child" has become a joke and cliché in our culture and that's unfortunate, but the Master said that "unless you change and become like little children you will never enter the kingdom of heaven" (Matthew 18:3). The kingdom of heaven is within, as is our inner child. Yours is probably sitting on her throne, yawning and waiting for you to come ask her out to play.

Your great celibacy adventure could take the form of doll collecting, tap dancing, or white water rafting! Maybe you feel compelled to read self-help books or join a yoga class. Wherever your adventure takes you, go with the flow! Have fun!

If yours was not a great childhood, that's okay. You can mother your inner child, raise her, and love her the way you should have been loved when you were a girl. A woman in my doll-making class told me a story that makes this point beautifully. When she was fourteen years old, her mother confiscated all her Barbie dolls and gave them away. Apparently, she was "too old" to be playing with dolls. She was devastated. She loved her Barbies. Not only did the act drive a wedge between her and her mother, she got the erroneous message that playtime was over and it was time to "grow up." She, like so many of us, learned to redefine play as romance and, later, sex. After many years of soul-searching, my classmate has finally given herself permission to play with Barbies. She does their hair and makes them beautiful clothes.

Come out and play! Like Mama always said, you need some fresh air!

PLAY 101. If you're not used to playing, you might not know how to start, what to try. One of the best places to start is your childhood. So get out your journal and get to writing.

♦ When you were a girl, what was a good time for you? Think back and record your favorite activities in a photocopy of the space below or your journal.

_____

_____

_____

✦ Write about one experience from your childhood that was so much fun you can remember every delicious moment. What were you doing? Who were you playing with? How old were you? Write it down.

_____

_____

_____

✦ Try to recall a fun time (not sexual) that you experienced as an adult. What were you doing? Who were you playing with? Write it down. (If you can't think of anything, make up something. Your imagination can help you discover what you'd like to be doing.)

_____

_____

_____

Now choose an activity from your list of childhood favorites and commit to doing it this week. Every week, try something new. Eventually you will discover a play activity that makes you laugh and gives you joy. Please do not skip this step. If your term of celibacy feels like work, you're going to end up looking for any human with a penis. Use your time alone to find out what makes you happy. If you know what that is, then go do it!

> *I was a virgin till I was twenty, then again till I was twenty-three.*
>
> —CARRIE SNOW

Self-discovery is a lifelong process. So far I've gone roller-skating (too rough on the knees now), biking (loved it!), and tap dancing (loved it!). I took my daughter to an amusement park recently and to my dismay, almost threw up on the Tilt O'Whirl. I guess there are some things I can't do anymore, but the great news is, I've got the rest of my life to figure it all out!

If after doing the above exercises, you still can't think of ways to have fun, here are some suggestions to jump-start your search:

✦ Throw a party with lots of loud music and food. Only invite the most fun, outrageous party animals. Hire a comic, and laugh and dance the night away.

✦ When was the last time you played cards or a board game with a friend? Remember Twister? Wouldn't that be a great adults-only co-ed party (but remember your Celibacy Promise!)?

✦ Join a sports team—bowling, softball, volleyball, etc., are great fun, and you get some exercise to boot.

✦ One of the Park District recreational centers in my town gives a water aerobics class for seniors. I crashed it and had too much fun. I had to work hard to keep up!

✦ In fact, search out recreational events for active seniors in your area. If they let you in, you'll have a great time. Seniors who are full of the joy of life can teach us stressed-out younger women a thing or two about having fun.

✦ Are you the adventurous type but can't get away? Chances are you haven't explored your town and its surrounding areas. Do some research and find out about some of the best nature spots, bicycle paths, amusement parks, shopping districts, etc.

✦ Many of us passionate women have big appetites for food. In fact, for better or worse, we tend to eat more for enjoyment than survival. Take a cooking class. Discover new restaurants. Try out a new ethnic recipe. Your area might even have a singles supper group. Go join today, or start one.

✦ Remember how for hours and hours we could jump rope without getting tired? Grab a couple of girlfriends, a rope, and jump some double Dutch. This could be a fun alternative to aerobics class.

A couple of months after my daughter was born, I had the great fortune to meet a wonderful woman who agreed to baby-sit so that I could go back to work. This woman was in her late fifties, but had the energy of a twenty-year-old. She loved children. While I barely had enough energy for my newborn, she easily kept up with the four babies and toddlers in her care. Her secret? She had an upbeat, positive attitude and no matter what the crisis, she laughed a lot, and *she liked to play.* Every week she bowled and played bid whist. Once or twice a year, she and her husband traveled, often to play in Las Vegas. The moral of the story? It's never too late to start playing and enjoying life.

Identify, Then Manage, Your Sexual Triggers

> *There are a number of mechanical devices which increase*
> *sexual arousal, particularly in women. Chief among them is*
> *the Mercedes-Benz 380SL convertible.*
>
> —P. J. O'Rourke

Of all the steps in this program, identifying and managing your sexual triggers—especially the managing part—is the most challenging. But the greatest challenge in a celibate's life is her greatest opportunity for fun.

A sexual trigger is anything that makes a woman want to do the wild thing. Earthy women practicing celibacy must become aware of the subtle and not-so-subtle situations, scenarios, and circumstances that turn them on, lest they accidentally end up in a man's apartment and his penis lands in her vagina. No more "accidental" or "it just happened" sex. Nine times out of ten, sexual encounters are premeditated anyway.

Earthy women have a vast repertoire of triggers. For example, before I knew myself and learned to love myself, I was highly susceptible to flattery. Because I didn't know for myself that I was a wonderful woman, I was totally dependent on men to tell me. And when they did, I'd instantly feel a rush of warmth. If you've ever fallen for any of the following lines, then flattery is probably a sexual trigger for you:

+ Hey, baby, you sure are fine.

+ You look really good in that dress.

+ You're not like other women I've met before. You're different.

+ It's really hard finding quality women like yourself.

+ You are a really intelligent woman.

A couple of months ago, I had to buy a new car, so my sisters and I went to a dealer. Would you believe that to cinch the deal, the salesguy resorted to flattery? "And let me just say," he said, "I hope you don't take this the wrong way, but you sisters are different from most of the women who come in here. I mean, I don't meet a lot of intelligent women." Laura, who had been snoozing during the negotiations, suddenly woke up. Janice, who is wary of everything and everyone, gave him one of her best withering looks. I liked the car, and he didn't have to go through all that. I knew we were being handed a line, but what the salesguy didn't know was that he was absolutely right. We are different. We are intelligent. We are special—just like every other woman on the planet.

I thanked him, smiled sweetly, and got a few more bucks knocked off the price of the car.

One of the most challenging tests of celibacy is learning to live with and enjoy erotic, passionate feelings that have not been dissipated through sexual intercourse or masturbation. A woman once told a gathering of churchwomen that when she is kissed by a man, her legs immediately fly open. We may not need a man for financial security or to fix a car, but we sure do love the pillow talk, romantic dinners, and touchy feely. Increasing the diversity of your play activities should help. Making your life a pleasure is your responsibility, not a man's.

In fact, one good way to determine if a man is good for you is to note whether or not you can have fun with him outside the bedroom. If the only good times you share are sexual, then you are both denying yourselves a greater, more fulfilling experience. For couples, a great side benefit of exploring the other bands of the play spectrum together is a heightened enjoyment of sex.

There are as many sexual triggers as there are women in the world, and every woman is different. One woman's turn-on may be another's wet blanket. For passionate women, however, any excuse for a thrill!

Close your eyes and think back to your most satisfying sexual experience. It may be difficult, but try not to get lost in feelings, sensations, and images. Instead, try and remember the steps that led up to the act. What did your partner do to turn you on so? Did he wear a certain fragrance or did he call you up the night before in that deep, sexy voice of his? Or was there something else—a haunting melody in the background, candlelight flickering?

As you analyze the event for any and all triggers, categorize them into one of the following groups: sight, taste, sound, touch, smell, and intuition (i.e., your psychic connection to a man). The more you are able to categorize your triggers, the better you'll recognize and understand your vulnerabilities. Write it all down in your journal.

I use the word "vulnerabilities" deliberately. In a healthy, happy, loving, monogamous, committed relationship (like marriage), playing with sexual triggers helps keep the love alive and the fire burning. However, in your celibacy practice, sexual triggers can be a death knell. They can throw a woman off her path and make her "forget" her promise to herself. Some triggers operate just below the threshold of consciousness, so if you don't know what yours are, you run the risk of being manipulated by them.

> *MAKE IT A POLICY NEVER TO HAVE SEX BEFORE THE FIRST DATE.*
>
> —SALLY FIELD, IN THE 1987 MOVIE *SURRENDER*

Weather, food, flattery, certain textures, art, music, dancing, laughing, and conversation can all serve as aphrodisiacs. It's important for a woman to know what her triggers are for two reasons:

+ *Awareness.* How many of us have said, "I don't know how it happened, but the next thing I knew, we were having sex." If you know you're not ready to have sex but can be easily tempted (oh, you earthy woman), it is crucial to know what your triggers are so that you can prevent "accidentally" falling into bed with a man.

✦ *Self-Discovery.* If you know what triggers your sexual and sensual feelings, then you can begin to consciously apply them to romancing yourself and expanding your awareness of the possibilities inherent in the play spectrum.

As you can see, this step is extremely important if you are serious about your promise to practice celibacy for a time. In fact, bringing your sexual triggers up to the level of conscious awareness will be one of the most important exercises you'll do to strengthen your celibacy practice. For example, every year when spring rolls around I feel the need to make a baby. Why? Because spring is my mating season. Any change in season produces sexual feelings in me. The change from hot to cold makes me want to cuddle. The first days of autumn make me want to cuddle. Here are some more of my favorite triggers:

Romantic, trashy novels

Certain times of the day, week, month, year (including holidays)

My birthday

Certain textures (mink, silk, etc.)

Engagement rings

Incense

Grey Flannel cologne

Jazz music (heavy on the sax)

Memories of erotic adventures

A man's deep and sexy baritone voice

Erotic dreams

Eating a meal with a man

My successes, my failures

Penetrating gazes

Dancing

Laughing

A man's touch

A man's attention

Crying

The sight of a tall, dark, thick man

Full moon

Champagne

Sunsets, sunrises

When I'm in a relationship, the triggers make sense. When I'm alone, the triggers will leave me feeling frustrated, depressed, and lonely if I don't manage them. So what I've learned to do is convert many of the triggers into self-love activities, and in the chart on page 126, that's what you're going to do. This exercise should help you expand your awareness and tap into the vastness of the play spectrum. If you can convert even a few triggers, you will be well on your way to making your celibacy practice a fun, rich time. I offer you my conversion chart as an example, but by all means, be creative. Tap into your growing self-knowledge base to convert the triggers into meaningful solo activities. As you go through your list, you'll notice that not all triggers should be converted. For example, I don't want to do anything about my response to a man's baritone voice or the Grey Flannel he wears or his tall, thick body!

How would you answer the following question: "Would you be content to be held close and treated tenderly and forget about the 'the act'? Answer Yes or No." The nationally syndicated newspaper columnist Ann Landers posed this question to her readers in the mid-'80s.

Apparently Ann touched a nerve; she received 100,000 replies in four days. *Seventy-two percent* said all they wanted was touching, no sex.

Ann's survey may not have been scientifically conducted, but a response of 100,000 is worth a look. If touching and holding is what most women crave, we can get that from most anyone! Women practicing celibacy from coast to coast should be rejoicing. Children are great huggers, as are family members, good friends, and new friends. Hug yourself! Women practicing celibacy need *at least* ten good full-body hugs every day, so hug a lot, and hug with abandon.

Now fill in a copy of the conversion chart of your top six sexual triggers.

*M*Y MOST MEMO-RABLE "ONSCREEN" SEX SCENE CAME TO BE MY MOST TREASURED FANTASY. IT WAS ON THE BEACH IN *FROM HERE TO ETERNITY* WITH BURT LANCASTER AND DEBORAH KERR. THE WAY IN WHICH THE TWO LOVERS MET AND HELD THEIR CELIBACY UNTIL THE VERY END OF THE FILM CREATED A SEXUAL TENSION AND FRUSTRATION AMONG THE VIEWERS, MYSELF INCLUDED. THE IMAGE OF THE TWO FINALLY COMING TOGETHER IN THE END ON THE WHITE SANDS, WITH THE OCEAN CRASHING OVER THEM, CREATED THE PURRR-FECTLY TIME-LESS SCENE.

—EARTHA KITT

SEXUAL TRIGGERS	CONVERSIONS TO SOLO ACTIVITIES
✦ *Romantic movies and trashy novels.*	Watch romantic comedies. They satisfy the craving for romance but don't take love and romance too seriously. Make you laugh about relationships and all the craziness that can go with them.
✦ *Times of the day, week, month, year.* The times when I feel sexiest are at the end of the day, Fridays and Saturdays, when I'm ovulating, holidays, and change of seasons.	Create self-love rituals for those times when you're at your most sensual. For example, at the end of the day, take a bubble bath with jazz music playing in the background. Take deep belly breaths. Buy new soft bed linens as winter ends and spring begins.
✦ *Birthdays.* When I'm in a relationship, I love for my man to lavish attention and gifts on me.	Mail a funny, outlandish birthday card to yourself. Buy yourself flowers or a new outfit. Forgive all your trespasses against yourself. Celebrate the gift of your life with balloons and confetti. Throw yourself a surprise birthday party. A musician friend of mind did that and 200 of his closest friends came to celebrate with him. It was one of the sweetest things he's ever done for himself.
✦ *Erotic dreams.* These dreams are so real that waking up is usually a big disappointment.	Upon awakening, savor the sensations, remember the details. This dream is one for your journal. Next, describe the man in your dreams. What did he look like? What did he do to turn you on so? Now for the rest of the day, recall

the dream in your private moments and be grateful for this gift. If the man in your dream was the kind of man you'd like to know in real life, bring him out of that realm and make him real. Remember him. Write a letter to him. Draw him in your journal. Remember the characteristics you loved most about him so that you can recognize them when Mr. Right enters your life.

♦ *Penetrating gazes. Ooo-wee,* when a man looks at me with that gaze, I turn into a powder puff.

Look at yourself in the mirror. Make sure the area is well lit. Stare at your beautiful eyes, the shape of your nose, your lovely lips. Smile at yourself. You might feel silly at first, but do it anyway. No one is watching. Now say, "I love you. You are an incredible woman." You might be tempted to look away, but hold your gaze. This is a powerful self-love exercise.

♦ *Touch.* A beloved's touch sends electricity through my body.

Touch and hug your friends. Hug your child, your mother, father, siblings. Hug yourself. When you are introduced to a new person, don't shake hands (although that's better than nothing), hug them. Can you imagine how boardrooms across America would change for the better if corporate execs started hugging?

SEXUAL TRIGGERS	CONVERSION TO SOLO ACTIVITIES
1. _____	_____
_____	_____
_____	_____
2. _____	_____
_____	_____
_____	_____
3. _____	_____
_____	_____
_____	_____
4. _____	_____
_____	_____
_____	_____
5. _____	_____
_____	_____
_____	_____
6. _____	_____
_____	_____
_____	_____

Masturbation

When I first began using the phrase "sensual celibacy," many people thought I was talking about masturbation. Old perceptions die hard, and because celibacy has long been viewed as a prudish lifestyle, it's difficult to convince folks that a woman practicing celibacy can still feel sexy, romantic, and passionate—and that's not masturbation. That's living.

Masturbation is a difficult topic for me to talk about because my parents are still alive. (My mother still thinks that masturbation will make you blind and crazy.) Seriously, masturbation is so intensely personal that I hate to bring it up, but it is an important issue for passionate women practicing celibacy, so I've got to address it. I believe that women should not engage in excessive masturbation. I know the word "excessive" is loaded. How much is excessive? Once a day? Twice a week? Five times a day? Once a month? Who's to say what's excessive? My concern is not how many times you do it (although five times a day *may* signal a problem that you might want to check out with a therapist). Masturbation can undermine one of the goals of the Sensual Celibacy Program, which is learning how to love and live comfortably with erotic feelings and using those earthy feelings to feel romantic about the self, nature, life's work, and so on. A woman gains strength when she can feel horny and simply enjoy the feeling.

That said, of course celibate people, women and men, will masturbate from time to time. The sex surveys and studies reveal that most women do it. It's a good way for a woman to know her own body and to make herself feel good. Sex with a man is the ultimate, but self-pleasuring can do in a pinch. One woman told me that before going out on a date, she masturbates. That way she's not tempted to fall into her date's bed and accidentally have sex. For this woman, masturbation is a way to strengthen her celibacy practice and keep her promise to herself (remember your Celibacy Promise?).

Monitor the content of your fantasies. Like the Master said, we are gods, and one of the formulas of creation is Fantasies + Sexual Energy = Manifestation. Let's not forget how powerful we are. We have the power to create with our mind, will, and energy, and our creations begin with a thought. In the physical, sexual energy leads to babies. In the etheric realm, sexual energy combined with repetitive fantasy can lead to spiritual and psychological babies. This can work either for or against us, depending on what we're visualizing. If you visualize yourself with a lot of money while you are in the throes of orgasm, who knows? Maybe you'll win the lottery.

Rape and bondage fantasies are a different story. They may be titillating for some women and some schools of thought believe that it is okay to let our minds roam in these shadowy realms, but I think this kind of fantasy could be dangerous to a woman's emotional health and serve to reinforce her attraction to really bad boys.

Remember our discussion about having sex while feeling guilty or ashamed and how that harms our souls? The same holds true for masturbating while feeling ashamed or guilty. Those of us with strict upbringings may have been made to feel guilty about touching ourselves. Intellectually we may be open and modern, but deep down there may be ambivalence. Don't keep going on automatic. Stop and sort out your feelings about it. Seek help if you feel it has become a problem. If your religion prohibits you from masturbating and you agree with this, then don't do it. The long-term guilt will overwhelm the short-term pleasure.

A final thought about self-pleasuring: Some people feel that if you masturbate, you are not practicing celibacy. The technical component of my definition of celibacy is "no penile penetration." Thus, I believe that a woman can masturbate and still remain celibate. As in all things, though, let your conscience be your guide.

Bedwork Assignments

The bedroom of a single woman says more about her hopes
and ambitions than any other space in her home.

—Marlene Adler Marks ("Bed of Roses,"
Living Fit, March 1997, p. 124)

In the essay "Bed of Roses," Marlene Adler Marks tells the poignant story of her relationship to her bed after her husband died.

The memories stored in my mattress at home were rooting me down. Each sag and crevice memorialized our marriage; a huge indentation on the right side recalled with perfection where my husband used to lie. It had been years since we had slept together, but each night, unconsciously, I let even the bed frame keep him alive for me.

Adler Marks reclaimed her relationship to her bed by buying an all new bed wardrobe. I've done something as simple as flipping over the reversible comforter. Now that your bed is your own again, you need to go through the process of reclaiming it. You need to feel comfortable in it by yourself. The following activities will help you and your bed become friends again.

In 114 b.c. a temple was dedicated to Venus Verticordia (Venus, Turner of Hearts) to celebrate the acquittal of two of the Vestal Virgins who had been accused of breaking their vows of celibacy. But any priestess found guilty suffered a horrible fate—she was ceremonially walled up alive in a small chamber beneath the city walls.

—A. T. Mann and Jane Lyle, *Sacred Sexuality*

✦ How is your bed dressed now that you're celibate? Plain old white sheets? Did you even make up your bed this morning? The bed is an important tool of sexual lovemaking, and we tend to neglect it when there's no man in our life. Make sure that you make up your bed every morning as soon as you wake up. Buy sheets in colors that make you feel romantic and alive, and textures that feel soft and silky on the skin (satin and Egyptian cottons are wonderful).

✦ Is your bed half empty or half full? Your bed is not half empty. It is not even half full. Your bed is filled to overflowing with your delectable self.

How do you sleep in your bed? Do you sleep in the middle of the bed or on the edge? I tend to sleep on the edge, as if keeping the other side ready and waiting for a man. Look, if you insist on viewing celibacy as a state of loss or emptiness, you're going to make yourself miserable. Stop looking over at the other side of the bed and patting the pillow in longing and despair. Claiming your bed is an important exercise for coming to terms with, making peace with, and wholeheartedly accepting your solitude and celibacy practice.

Tonight, before you go to sleep, assess your position on the bed. Where are you? Are you on the edge, about to fall off? If so, ease your way to the middle of the bed. This may feel uncomfortable, but force yourself to stay put. When I first started this exercise, I'd often have to back butt first into the middle of the bed.

Once you're in the middle of the bed, lay flat on your back and stretch your arms and legs so that, as much as possible, they reach to the four corners of your bed. Now roll back over to the edge of the bed. Now roll roll roll over to the other side. If your bed's strong enough, jump up and down! Play! It's your bed. Practice filling up your bed space every night for a week or two.

As you stretch and roll, repeat the following affirmation (or make up one of your own):

AFFIRMATION: *I am a beautiful, sensual woman who just happens to be practicing celibacy for a time. I claim my bed. I stake my territory. I love my time alone.*

CHAPTER EIGHT

Step 6—
Mind Your Body

*Inside this fat body there's a skinny person screaming
to get out. How'd she get in there? I ate her.*

—Anonymous

What an amazing vehicle we've been given to accomplish our work here on earth. Not only does it move us around from here to there, it gifts us with myriad sensual pleasures. The body is an integrated composition of 206 bones, about 5 quarts of blood, 72 heartbeats per minute, 100 trillion cells, 10 billion nerve cells, and 700 voluntary muscles. Your network of capillaries equals about 1.5 acres.

Deepak Chopra's *Ageless Body, Timeless Mind* forever changed the way we view the human body. According to Chopra, that old sack of blood and bones is really a quantum field of ever changing information. Atoms, the building blocks of our bodies and all life, are composed of "99.9999 percent empty space!" Why then are American woman plagued by diseases and ailments of every hue and stripe if we're only empty space? According to Chopra and many other thinkers, researchers, and physicians, we get sick and age because we expect to.

An impressive multidisciplinary body of research has emerged during the latter decades of this century testifying to the mind-body-soul interconnection. Your thoughts and emotions directly affect your body's health. If you are repressed, feel hopeless about life, and are unable to express your emotions, you're at risk. This is how celibacy used to be practiced. Repression has been the accepted method of dealing with unruly sexual passions. Old-style celibate women suffer in silence, rebound with men in fear, feel hopeless about their marital prospects, and are often angry at their ex-partners. Needless to say, this approach is unhealthy. It's no mystery to me that incidences of breast and other cancers, as well as many other stress-related illnesses, in women have been rising right alongside escalating divorce rates.

Concepts like forgiveness, gratitude, and celebrating sensuality are cornerstones of the Sensual Celibacy Program. I'm not exaggerating when I say that working this Program could save your life!

More than any other group, women practicing celibacy must learn not only to tend their bodies, but feel good about their bodies. During this current Celibacy Period 6, I have set as my number one priority getting my body in shape. I am improving my overall health and energy levels through diet, exercise, and stress-reduction techniques.

During both of my pregnancies, I gained a lot of weight. The body that I wear today was created during my first pregnancy and "blossomed" during my second. Although it's not unusual for a woman to gain weight and keep it on after she's had children, it can be unhealthy, and research is showing that the loss of even a few pounds can produce health benefits. Obesity has been linked to all sorts of ailments, including heart disease, some cancers, and diabetes. Without a doubt, all that extra weight takes a toll on a woman's body. Combine that with the daily stresses of life and you've produced a time bomb that could explode into a heart attack, stroke, ulcer, or any number of physical ailments.

ARBIE AND KEN PROBABLY HAVE THE RECORD FOR THE LONGEST-STANDING CELIBATE RELATIONSHIP. I'M SURE THEY'D LIKE TO HAVE SEX, BUT THEY CAN'T.

My personal celibacy timeline dramatically illustrates how relationship stresses directly coincided with setbacks in my attempts to lose weight. Every time I started to make progress in losing weight and firming up, I would allow relationship stress to not only stop me, but reverse my progress. For example, during Celibacy Period 3, I gave up sugar and coffee, fasted for ten days, gave up all meat (including poultry and fish), and exercised. I was losing weight and feeling great. I met Father #2, got pregnant, became a meat eater again (i.e., poultry and fish), and gained more weight than ever before. That was not his fault, but mine.

Men are constantly trying to give me advice on how to lose weight, and in trying to please them, I've listened. One told me to eat only raw vegetables. He said, "I've never dated anyone with a weight problem before." What a nice thing to say. Another told me to eat only one meal a day (I thought I was going to die). In the relationship following Celibacy Period 5, the man constantly told me, "Donna, if you lose the weight, I'll marry you tomorrow" or "Donna, if you lose the weight, I'll buy you a ring." Wow, what incentive. So I powerwalked every day and ate low-fat foods. I actually lost fifteen pounds, and I was too pleased with myself. The only problem was that as the relationship started to disintegrate, the weight crept back on—all fifteen pounds, plus five more. The moral of my story: *Get your body in shape for yourself!*

Now I'll admit, I'm not a little woman, but I'm not a mountain either. No, I do not conform to the Barbie mold, but I don't know any woman who does—not even thin women. To use this period of celibacy to get my body in shape *for me* is a supreme act of self-love.

Most of us have a few pounds to lose, but the goal should be freedom from food issues forever. That means you've got to start digging around in your past again to find out what old, obsolete subconscious programs have been keeping you in bondage to brownies and french fries.

Heaviness can serve us well. If your size makes you feel unattractive, it is "protecting" you from men (which is impossible since, even with the extra pounds, you are an attractive woman). In her book *Why Weight? A Guide to Ending Compulsive Eating*, Geneen Roth says that "compulsive eating is *always* an attempt to care for yourself." If weight is one of your big issues, use this period of celibacy to make a concerted effort to pay attention to how you use food to escape from uncomfortable emotions. The big secret of naturally thin women is that they too have issues; theirs just don't show up on the body. Whatever your health and body image issues are, use this time to deal with them.

Why is celibacy such a good time to improve your health and deal with body issues? No men! At least not looking at your naked body in your bedroom. It's not so much that men are supercritical of our bodies, although some men have a lot of nerve. It's our perception of how men appreciate the feminine body that contributes to the breakdown in communication and understanding. We see them lusting after *Playboy* models, and we think that's what they want. They make a lot of noise about other women's body parts, and of course ours don't measure up. Our perceptions—not what a man says or does—create our self-esteem. Apart from telling a man that you don't appreciate his lusting after other women, you can't control what anyone says or does, but you can control how you feel and respond to comments and actions.

I've also heard women complain that their men won't support them in a weight-loss effort. At every turn they are being seduced into eating all kinds of junk that they shouldn't. Unless the man is forcing the food down your throat, which he isn't, then this excuse is just that, an excuse.

Yes, it would be nice if he would help, but ultimately, you are responsible for your own behavior.

Many, many men have told me that thinness, or heaviness for that matter, is not the ideal. Men are visual creatures, but when they look at you, they are checking out the entire package. Not just your big thighs, but your long eyelashes and pretty smile. They look at how you carry yourself. They listen to the quality of your voice and the integrity or humor of your words. Yes, men can be difficult, but I think we underestimate their ability to love us, regardless of whether we're a size 6 or a size 18.

I don't have the statistics to prove it, but based on the experiences of my friends, as well as my own, single mothers are a particularly high-risk group for all sorts of obesity and stress-related ailments. And even the most positive, energetic single moms I know succumb to bouts of depression and low self-esteem from time to time.

Single mothers who are not in relationships and who are practicing celibacy should beware the risks of misplacing their feminine identity, which directly influences body image. Typically, a single mom's entire life revolves around work and children. Little attention is given to socializing (kiddie birthday parties and school assemblies don't count) and pampering. We come up with all sorts of excuses, from no time to no money, but the truth is, we're worn out from the stress and maybe a little scared of stepping back out into the world. My friend Dawn says that she always counsels single mothers to take vacations away from their children. (She told me this just as she was leaving for two weeks in Hawaii.)

All women practicing celibacy must find creative, healthy ways to regularly celebrate their sexuality and sensuality. You'll know that the Program is working when you no longer need the extra pounds to protect you from men. You're learning to trust in your ability to make good, well-informed decisions about the men in your life—about all areas in your life.

If getting your health together doesn't motivate you to start a food and exercise program, then think about how good you'll look in cute clothes. Use your vanity to get the job done.

When was the last time you felt good, with your energy level high, no aches and pains? Now how do you feel today? Are you at optimum health, or are you just faking it? The mind-body connection is real. Even Western science is finally admitting that our thoughts and emotions have an impact on the health of our body.

All women, whether practicing celibacy or sexually involved, have stress in their lives, and thus are at risk for a whole host of ailments. Some researchers are saying that as much as 85 percent of diseases are stress related. The good news is that stress-related diseases are wholly preventable.

Are you doing anything about the stress in your life, or are you pushing your body to the limit? I made that mistake during my ill-fated relationship following Celibacy Period 5. I was so stressed out with what was going on that I missed two months of my menstrual cycle. For women who tend to be irregular, that may not be such a big deal, but for an extremely regular woman like me, missing two months was cause for alarm. In addition, my blood pressure shot up forty points.

My kindly old-school doctor didn't just poke and prod and pre-scribe pills. He asked me what was going on in my life. As I told him, tears stung my eyes. I knew my relationship was bothering me, but what I hadn't factored in was my job layoff a few months prior, my part-time consulting job, raising two children as a single parent, trying to run a company, and a book deadline. After I finished the long list, my doctor said, "If I were your period, I wouldn't show up either."

As to marriage or celibacy, let a man take the course he will. He will be sure to repent.
—Socrates

The body-mind connection is real, and if you value your health, you won't let anything or anyone prevent you from being your healthy best. Properly caring for and feeding the body is as important to your well-being as nourishing the soul. Without health, the quality of life is reduced. Without a healthy appreciation for your body, regardless of your size or shape, you'll probably continue to mistreat it with junk food, alcohol, tobacco, drugs, and casual sex.

Any good body-renovation project should be comprised of the following four components: exercise, proper nutrition, stress reduction, and a healthy body image.

EXERCISE. In *Sister Feelgood,* I promoted the idea that exercise should be fun. No more "working out." We human beings are drawn to activities that give us pleasure (like sex) and are repelled by those that produce pain.

There's been a lot of talk on the news lately about all the weight Americans are gaining—despite the research, books, exercise gadgets, weight-loss programs, and gurus on the market. En masse, we are rebelling against the idea of more work. Moreover, all that jumping around in high-impact aerobics classes is bad for the joints. I think low-impact aerobics came on the scene just one heartbeat too late.

However, the fact still remains that a sedentary lifestyle promotes weight gain, which can become a health problem. No movement makes the joints stiff and the circulation sluggish. Our metabolism goes to sleep. We need to get moving, but before you go out and buy yet another health club membership or piece of exercise equipment take the time to find an activity that you will actually enjoy. Here's a list of my personal favorites:

tap dancing, belly dancing, freestyle dancing

roller-skating

walking, hiking

tennis

swimming

biking

sex (oh, well)

Any good exercise program will focus on strength, flexibility, and endurance. For strength, I do exercises in which I can use my own weight as resistance (e.g., push-ups). I also use dumbbells. Yoga keeps me flexible (if I do it every day), so much so that I feel as if I've received a full-body massage. For my endurance activity, I walk or do low-impact aerobics about forty minutes a day, four or five days a week. And whenever possible, I dance and swim.

Lack of motivation and time seem to be the biggest barriers to consistency, so I'll tell you what I do to prevent excuse making. For motivation, I use music to charge up my walk. The combination of movement, good music, and beautiful scenery makes me high. It feels so good. After my walk, I do about 100 sit-ups using my abdominal cruncher. Yes, I did buy a gadget, but I love how it works. While I'm doing my sit-ups, I watch exercise shows on ESPN. Although I have no desire to buff up, the high fitness levels of the instructors, male and female, give me incentive to keep going.

I also pray during my routines—especially during yoga (I thank my God after successfully completing each asana, because for me to get through one of those postures is truly a miracle), and I often pray during my walks.

As for not being able to exercise because of lack of time, I've used that excuse too. But if I'm going to be completely honest with myself, I'll have to admit that during the course of a day, I have probably let many opportunities to exercise pass me by. Exercise is such a loving thing to do for the body that has given you so much pleasure, you've got to make time, even if it means getting up a half hour before children wake up or going to bed a half hour later to get your routine in later in your day.

No matter what your current fitness level or size, you can start exercising today. Check with your doctor first, but I don't think she'll have a problem with your walking around the block for starters. Gradually increase your time and pace, and you'll be fine-tuning your metabolism to work efficiently on behalf of your weight-loss goals. Don't expect immediate results. Healing your body and changing your lifestyle take time, but are well worth the effort.

A final thought for women practicing celibacy: During those times when the horniness is at a feverish pitch, exercise is a great "quick fix" way to calm down your hormones. Exercise shakes off excess energy.

Paradoxically, depending on the types of exercise you do, certain movements can also stir up sexual feelings. Women who have been in the celibate mode for a year or more will find that as hormonal levels subside, so may sexual desire. This is a great blessing—except for those times when you want to just remember what desire feels like. An exercise known as the pelvic tilt will stir up the lower regions, as well as the memories. *For Advanced Celibates Only:* Simply lie on your back with knees raised, feet flat on the floor. Now slightly and gently, lift your hips up and off the floor. When you raise your hips, do a Kegel clench. Mercy! The image of your hips going up and down is a beautiful sight to behold. Turn on the music, get a rhythm going, and your "workout" will take you to a new level of experience. *(Do not do this exercise if you have not yet learned how to enjoy sexual feelings without having to have sex.)*

PROPER NUTRITION. There are so many diets being promoted and so much research-based information, some of which conflicts, that I hesitate to prescribe any program. Instead, I encourage you to do some research on your own. Our bodies may have the same basic design, but no two are alike. We all have different dietary requirements. One woman's high-carbohydrate food program may cause another to feel restless, irritable, and sleepy. You may not be temperamentally suited to a low-fat diet, while a program of traditionally prepared foods eaten in moderation might work for you.

The following are my laywoman's recommendations for a healing diet:

+ *Cut the fat,* but not entirely. We need some fat in our diet, so don't be afraid of it. Some diet regimens prescribe as low as ten grams of fat per day. I can't imagine living like that. Twenty-five to thirty grams per day might be more reasonable.

+ *Cut the salt,* but not entirely (unless your doctor says so). We all need salt for healthy functioning, but processed foods are usually way too high in sodium content. Women prone to bloating will see a definite improvement.

+ *Don't eat fake food.* I know a woman who is so stressed about losing weight that she has no real food in her refrigerator. Everything is a chemical. Fake butters, sugars, salts, flavor enhancers (MSG—bad, bad), and even fats abound on your grocer's shelves, but stay away from them. Instead, eat real foods that are healthily prepared. Learn new cooking techniques (no more frying) so that your food is naturally low in fat, flavorful, and healthy. It is possible.

✦ *Drink a lot of water.* If you hate drinking water, then eight glasses a day is going to be a hardship and your diet has just become more work. Start out with one glass of water per day and build slowly. Squeeze some lemon or lime into the water (great for internal cleansing). Instead of drinking juices or sodas with your meals, drink water. I believe that teas qualify as water, although if you add sweetener, you've sort of defeated your purpose.

✦ *Cut a lot of the sugar.* Some people are fanatics about cutting out all sugars in their diet. Some have to be because of health issues, but if you're not bothered by problems such as hyperglycemia, then a little bit of sugar won't hurt. Everything in moderation.

✦ *Reduce your meat intake.* Meat is heavy. Even low-fat meat is heavier than other protein-rich foods such as eggs and beans. Meat is also harder to digest. Instead of making meat the centerpiece of your dinners, make it a side dish to veggies, beans, pasta, and rice.

✦ *Add fruits and veggies.* Five servings every day will hopefully keep the doctor away.

✦ *Add soy products* if you are menopausal. Researchers have found that Asian women have few associated symptoms (e.g., hot flashes) because their diets are high in soy products.

✦ *Take vitamin supplements* if you need to. Women are often low in iron and calcium. Check with your doctor first.

One of the many pleasures our body gives us is the ability to enjoy the taste of food. Nature could have made all our fruits and vegetables taste like rice cakes, but she didn't. Instead, we have been given a veritable taste banquet of food. For women who crave sensation, food can give us a little bit of heaven on earth.

One of the dangers of giving up a sensual experience (e.g., sex) is that we tend to try and compensate in other areas. Women who give up sex for a time often turn to food for comfort and excitement. Food is our friend and it doesn't talk back. Nourishment is the least of our concerns. We must learn to balance the appreciation for taste with the basic nutritional requirements of our bodies. We must learn to fearlessly confront uncomfortable emotions instead of using food to medicate them. I would highly recommend Geneen Roth's books (*Breaking Free from Compulsive Eating* and *Feeding the Hungry Heart*). Her work is compassionate and understanding of the emotional dependence so many women have on food.

The unsung heroes of our age are the chefs who are conjuring ingenious ways to cut the fat while retaining the flavor of our favorite foods. Dishes that have been traditionally off-limits to people trying to lose weight—for example, Mexican and soul food—have received complete and satisfying makeovers. No longer do we have to give up our favorite foods. We literally can eat anything we want, in moderation of course. This revelation and the self-knowledge you acquire from staying in touch with your emotions will greatly reduce your need to binge. If you need to binge, however, go ahead and binge. Just try and be intelligent about it. Don't go on automatic anymore. Stay conscious of the damage a high-fat binge will do to your program. Instead of eating bags and bags of potato chips, eat a ton of low-fat herb popcorn. For brownie attacks, there are no-fat brownie mixes available, and they make excellent brownies. Plop a scoop of some low-fat vanilla ice cream on top, and you'll be humming and tapping your feet, guilt-free.

What's your favorite dish? When was the last time you had a chance to enjoy it? I was raised on Jamaican food and I love ackee and codfish. Ackee is not always available, so when I get it, I'm in heaven.

Good food makes me happy. Earthy women usually have big appetites and enjoy eating hearty meals. Some women will not eat a full meal in front of a man, as if their big appetite will offend or make them feel less than a woman. So they'll pick at some plain lettuce and then binge like crazy when they get home.

Food has gotten such a bad rap recently with our national weight-loss obsession. As a society, we've developed a collective food fear. Don't deny yourself the sensual pleasure of eating good food. If you're losing weight, do some research on how to prepare your favorite dishes healthily and deliciously. Remember, for women practicing celibacy, the goal is to enjoy your sensuality, not suppress it.

STRESS REDUCTION. Stress is a lot like the weather: We talk a lot about it but we don't do anything to change it. Usually, it takes some crisis to make us realize that we need to manage the challenges in our life in better ways. Fortunately, there's a lot we can do, and it doesn't have to cost you anything.

Breathe. "I already breathe," I hear you saying, but if you're not inhaling from deep down in your diaphragm, you are not breathing deeply enough. Most of us breathe from within our chest. The more deeply you breathe, the more oxygenated your body will become. In *Jumpstart Your Metabolism,* Pam Grout goes so far as to suggest that breathing exercises can help us lose weight. Without a doubt, proper breathing stimulates energy and calms the mind. Get quiet, close your eyes, relax your shoulders. Now inhale for four counts, hold the breath for four counts, and exhale for eight counts. Put your hand on your tummy. If you're breathing correctly, your hand will rise with each inhalation and fall with each exhalation. With your very first diaphragmatic breath, you should feel a tangible difference in the activity level of the mind and the tension of the body. That's not to say that all thoughts will cease. They won't, at least not at first. For your first time out, just get used to the practice, and practice consistently for a few minutes every day.

Meditate. Breathing and meditation go hand in hand. As you breathe, notice how easily your body and mind relax in response. It's such a good feeling. First, pray for protection as you begin your journey inward. When you meditate, you become receptive to the still small Voice within. Your thoughts may flutter here and there, and that's okay. It takes consistent practice to quiet the noise of the mind. Just know that taking out even five minutes a day for yourself in this way heals mind, body, and soul.

Sit in nature. Those of us who live in the city don't touch trees and listen to birds nearly enough. Too much concrete, steel, and plastic can make life dreary, much like the mechanistic world of Big Brother in *1984*. Take the time to go outside, even in your own backyard, to stand on grass, put your hands in dirt. If you're feeling sad or lonely today, lay on the ground and let Mother Earth absorb your pain. If you're feeling happy, let the singing birds cheer you on. Nature heals us. We human beings were designed as an integral part of nature, and when we sit behind a computer or in front of a TV for too long, we feel completely out of our element. This can cause much stress. Go hug a tree today!

Take a mind vacation. Some of the best dreams are daydreams. Give yourself permission to let your mind soar to the Bahamas or the planet Venus. Tell the voice of that mean fifth-grade teacher who kept telling you to stop looking out of the window and pay attention to shut up and let you dream. If a daydream does not spontaneously come to you, I invite you to come fly with me:

VACATION 1

Take your mind to a faraway land of mists and mystery. You are a maiden dressed in a golden gossamer robe that barely conceals your mature, womanly body. It is a beautiful, warm, sunny day, and a gentle breeze kisses your skin. You stand in a wide open field containing flowers of many colors and sweet smells. The tiny bluebirds and sparrows sing soprano songs to you alone.

You walk through the field, the flowers brushing your legs with their soft, velvet petals, until you come to a stream of gently coursing clear, clean water. You dip your hand in, and happily, the water is warm. Slipping out of your robe, you step into the inviting water, which cleanses and refreshes your body. Swim and play in the water for as long as you like.

VACATION 2

You are in your private jet and are flying far from home. The pilot announces that you will reach your destination momentarily. In the meantime, you look down below, through the white, cottony clouds, to see ranges of snowcapped mountains.

The pilot gently lowers the plane on top of a mountain that is thick with trees and luscious green vegetation.

You are on the mountain now, steps away from a small temple. You remove your shoes and bow, then enter through the small wooden door. Inside the temple you are greeted by an old woman. You say, "Please help me. I was told that you already know my needs." She nods, then hands you a purple velvet bag tied with a string. She says, "Go back out the way you came. Climb to the highest point on this mountain; you only have a few more yards to go. Then open this bag and throw the contents out into the air, saying, 'I am healed. Thank God I am healed.' That is all." She returns to her duties and you go outside to do as she instructed.

You easily climb up the mountain until you reach the top. Opening the bag, you grab a handful of what feels like rocks and fling them out into the air. Hanging suspended in the air, the rocks turn into sparkles, like stars or glitter. You are in awe of the miracle and you clap your hands in delight. As the sparkles slowly fall to the earth, you see a vision. The sparkles are falling on you at work, on you with your man, on you with your children, and as they fall on you, they fall on all who come in contact with you.

After you empty the contents of the bag, you sit down. You feel happy and healed. Moreover, you know that from now on, all who come in contact with you will be healed too.

We all visualize and fantasize. The fantasies our minds easily create during sex are a good case in point. Our sexual fantasies further heighten our desire—a clear-cut example of the mind-body connection. Sexual fantasies can be dangerous for some celibates, but I bring them up because we all know their power well. If our fantasies can create sexual feeling in our bodies, then they can create other feelings as well—maybe even feelings that can cure our illnesses.

HEALTHY BODY IMAGE. If you've been working even a couple of steps of the Program, you should be getting a good idea of how your own values, behaviors, conditioning, and attitudes brought you to this point in your life.

I'm convinced that mirrors in clothing store fitting rooms add twenty pounds to your frame. Combine that with the bright, harsh lights, and I'm hiding from the mirror. I often experience the carnival mirror effect, i.e., it seems as if my body is being stretched and blown out of all proportion.

American women may come from different so-cial strata, races, religions, or geographical regions, but one thing most of us have in common is a nega-tive perception of our bodies. We feel we are too fat, too thin, too dark, too light, too short, too tall, too flat chested, too big breasted—and on and on. I don't know any woman who has made peace with her body—not one. That's not to say there are none, I just haven't met any.

We would start a revolution in America if, just for one day, we women would say to ourselves, "I love my body. My body is beautiful." I'm so tired of the media foisting impossible physical role models upon us. On the other hand, I don't have to accept them. Even at my thinnest, I was never a waif. Talk to a waif, and she'll probably express some dissatis-faction with her size too. Let's just say "enough is enough" and stop buying into the madness.

Mirror, mirror. I know you've heard this exercise a thousand times, but it's such a good one, I'm going to include it here. You know the drill: Take off your clothes and stand butt naked in front of a full-length mirror. (Keep the lights on!) Now assess your body. Is it really all that bad? Probably not. Now pretend you're posing for a pic-ture and smile at yourself. Smile seductively and arch your eyebrows. Tilt your head back and check out that gorgeous profile. Throw yourself a kiss and say, "You are one gorgeous woman!" and say it with as much positive loving emotion as you can muster.

Develop a walk. Have a friend help you assess your walk. Is it crisp and efficient, getting you from here to there? Does your posture make

> I'VE NEVER HAD A ONE-NIGHT STAND IN MY LIFE. . . . MY CRI-TERIA FOR HAVING SEX NOW IS, I HAVE TO BE DAMN NEAR IN LOVE WITH THE PERSON. IN FACT, I'VE RECENTLY DECIDED THAT I WOULDN'T BE HAVING SEX AGAIN UNTIL I'M MARRIED. . . . A GUY MIGHT BE ABLE TO SLOW ME DOWN, BUT HE'S NOT GOING TO BREAK ME. ANYTHING THAT PUTS ME IN TEMPTATION, I'M RE-SISTING.
>
> —TONI BRAXTON

you look tired or sad? I was told by a friend that I walked like my father. Of course, I was appalled, so I developed a new walk to convey and internalize confidence with a subtle touch of feminine sensuality. Here it is: First of all, *slow down!* Now lead with the breasts, slightly hold in the stomach, and swing your arms loosely and gracefully. You might want to add a signature movement. For example, I sometimes stretch out the pinky finger on my right hand. That's it. What's the point of developing a walk? The image that you present to the world says a lot about how you feel about yourself. If you walk as if the weight of the world is on your shoulders, you're probably feeling that way. If you just straighten up a bit, not only will you be perceived differently, but you'll feel better. Good posture helps the body's energy flow circulate more efficiently.

AFFIRMATION: *My body is beautiful. My body is healthy. I love my body. I thank God for my body.*

CHAPTER NINE

Step 7—
Get Out
of the House
and Mingle

Sheila said I'm too choosy, that my standards are too high, and because they seem nonnegotiable, she swears up and down that if I don't loosen up, the only person who'll ever meet my qualifications is God.

—Savannah, in Terry McMillan, *Waiting to Exhale*

✦ ✦ ✦

Have you ever jumped into a pool of water cold enough to take your breath away? Even inching your body into the water doesn't seem to ease the shock to your system. Only after you've been in the water awhile does your body become adjusted to the temperature and you begin to feel comfortable. The water doesn't change, you just feel better in it.

Dating after a long hiatus is a lot like jumping into a pool of freezing cold water. This pool of ever changing, bewildering rules and norms can be a shock to the system. The only way to become comfortable negotiating the dating scene is to get into the water—but you don't have to jump in all at once. Read this chapter first and ease your way in. Eventually you'll warm up and start having a lot of fun.

I loved how the excellent ensemble cast of *Seinfeld* depicted the dating scene. In their "love" relationships, the characters waded at the shallow end of the pool. Their relationships had the life span of a tsetse fly and about as much depth. They went from cute partner to cute partner, searching for what? Love? Their relationships fell apart every week, for any and all reasons, many of them bordering on the insane. Seldom did they dive into the deep end of the pool, the soul's love arena.

In many ways, dating is the same as it's always been. You meet a man. You go out to a movie, dinner, or dancing. You talk easily, or the conversation is strained. Either you like him or you don't. The questions in between are the ones that cause us so much anxiety: Should you go dutch or let him pay for everything? Should you let him kiss you or not? Should you have sex with him or not?

With AIDS and ever changing sexual roles, dating etiquette—what to say, how to say it, what to do, how to do it—can cause great anxiety

MOST PEOPLE HAVE HEARD THAT THE YOUNG CASANOVA WAS THE GREATEST ADVENTURER AND LOVER OF HIS TIME, BUT NOT MANY KNOW WHAT BECAME OF HIM. IN HIS LATER YEARS, HE LIVED IN BOHEMIA AND WORKED FOR COUNT VON WALDSTEIN IN THE CHATEAU DE DUX AS—OF ALL THINGS—A LIBRARIAN. THE RENOWNED LOVER PASSED AWAY QUIETLY IN THE STACKS, LEAVING MANY WOMEN DISAPPOINTED, NO DOUBT, AND MANY MEN RELIEVED.

—CHRISTINE SCHULTZ, *THE BOOK OF LOVE*

on both sides. Complicating the scene is your celibacy commitment. It's too bad there are no healthy images of women and men practicing celibacy on film or TV. Such images would help make the idea of romance and celibacy a comfortable, acceptable combination in the national consciousness. Some questions facing the abstaining woman are:

♦ Is it realistic to think that a woman can remain celibate while dating given her own healthy urges and external pressure to "give in"?

♦ Knowing that a woman is practicing celibacy, will a man agree to date her, or will he think spending money on flowers and romantic dinners is a waste of time?

♦ How does a man truly view a woman practicing celibacy? Does he respect her views, or is she a challenge to be conquered?

♦ At what point during courtship should a woman announce that she is practicing celibacy?

Practicing celibacy while dating today is like walking through a minefield; you don't know who's going to blow up when you announce that you're not having sex right now. Women have to be prepared for anything because anything can happen. The good news is that some aspects of dating will actually be simpler (though not necessarily easier). If at the beginning of your acquaintance you let a man know as a courtesy that you will not be having sex, then your position is clear. A decent man will respect you for telling him, and will either stick around or leave. He might choose to leave, and as painful as it might be at times, he has that right. Some men may be tolerant and understanding. As quiet as it's kept, not all men want sex right away. Many would just as soon wait awhile. Others may be furious, call you names (e.g., cocktease and bitch), then abruptly end the acquaintance.

And then there is the bad boy who may pretend to support your decision and even enter into a relationship with you. You think he's being celibate too, but he's got at least one backup plan, and her name is Suzie.

In addition, he may be viewing you as a challenge with the goal of getting you into bed. You'll find out his true intentions in one of two ways: (a) if you keep your promise to yourself and not have sex, or (b) if you break your promise to yourself and have sex with him. If you keep your celibacy promise, this type of man will eventually go away. If you break your promise to yourself and have sex with him, he will leave sooner.

Hold out for the good guys! Yes, they do exist and right in your own hometown. Keep your promise to yourself and hold off on sex as long as possible. If he stays and asks you to marry him and you actually walk down the aisle, then you've just been blessed with a special man. If you want this kind of man, you will have to be that kind of woman, not for him or anyone else but yourself.

Joyce was involved with a man who she thought had accepted and respected her stand on celibacy. Imagine her surprise and pain when, after a year of dating and deepening their relationship, he left. Her story has a happy ending, though. A couple of years later, she met another man who really did respect her decision. How did she know? She kept her promise to herself and he married her within a year.

How can a woman be sure of a man's commitment? I know it sounds archaic, but the only way a woman will know for sure is if he marries her! Although quality commitments can and do occur in relationships in which the partners are not married, no other contract besides marriage declares in such a public and legally binding way the love and commitment two people share. The cynics may object to this statement, citing the fact that half the couples that get married today get divorced. And it's true, divorce is a national epidemic. Still, most men do not enter into marriage lightly. This is the ultimate commitment to them, which they equate to a loss of freedom. For a man to even consider marriage speaks volumes about his love for a woman.

The divorce rate is high because people are marrying without resolving their individual issues first; they also haven't learned skills like communication and negotiation that are needed to keep a marriage strong. When we have sex too soon with a man, we lose perspective and objectivity because our focus is switched from couple work to play. How many times have you had sex with a man to make up after an argument, or had sex to avoid one? This is using play to avoid work, and in the long run, your relationship will suffer. In every relationship there is a time for play and a time for work. A balance of work and play helps to create and sustain a strong bond. However, all play and no work (and vice versa) will kill a relationship.

Women who jump into bed after hearing and making declarations of love might be mistaking horniness for love. A male friend of mine often says that "the level of intimacy two people have attained is frozen at the moment of sexual intercourse." Sex deepens the relationship only if true intimacy has been already achieved. Put another way, can a woman really have earth-shaking orgasms with a man she barely knows, likes, or trusts? If so, can that ecstasy be sustained over time?

Some women claim that sex for sex's sake is just fine. "He was just a fuck buddy, a maintenance man." Are you just some plumbing to be fixed or wires to be recircuited? Single women often advise one another to keep a man on the side for sexual emergencies until Mr. Right comes along. They say they can have sex and not care about the man, but I have yet to meet a woman for whom this is true. These women are in denial big time because when the man doesn't call or the man's other women become known, they're wild with pain and rage. They may not be in love, but their often violent reactions indicate that they do indeed have feelings for the man. At this point, things get very messy and soon they're on the Ricki Lake show crying, "But I have a man!"

Maybe there is one woman in the world who can have sex and not care about her partners, but she's not the norm and I wish we women would stop saying that and face the truth about ourselves. Is it so awful that we've been designed to *receive* and *retain* male energies and that most of us cannot have sex without having feelings for a man? What is so threatening about this idea, and why do we insist on disrespecting our unique design? Is it because our sex is not precious to us? Is it because our poverty and scarcity mentality has us believing that if we don't have sex with a man, he won't want us? Isn't the real reason for our denial *fear?* We adult women bemoan and lament the rise in teen pregnancies, but isn't their fear our fear too?

Sex too soon puts a relationship and your heart at risk. Sex delayed protects a newborn couple and gives you time to truly get to know a man.

If we neglect the care and feeding of our souls during dating by jumping into sex too soon, the loss feels that much more profound if we find ourselves alone again. Without another upon whom to heap our attention, we flinch at the first sight of celibacy, which is why it is so important to impart meaning and purpose to this special time in your life. If you don't, you'll soon be hunting for a man, any man, to fill the void.

About a year after the birth of my daughter and months after the breakup with her father, life threw me an interesting curve. An ex-boyfriend whom I'd not seen for many years came back into my life. Ours had been one of those intense karmic relationships with so many issues. We had never really succeeded in coming to terms with our different values, personalities, and life goals. We did have this tremendous sexual attraction, however, and despite all our differences, we truly cared about each other. Unfortunately, our love could not mask the problems caused by emotional immaturity on both of our parts. He was the leader, and I was the follower. I was the doormat, and he wore the shoes that were made for walking on doormats. I didn't have the faintest idea of who I was or what I wanted to do with my life. He was very clear about his goals. When we parted, I felt splintered into a million pieces.

Great spans of time passed, and I had healed, more or less, from that troubling relationship. When we met again, however, it was as if we had never parted. Although I was older, a little wiser, and committed to celibacy for a period, some things never change. We were still deeply attracted to each other, and the old, destructive pattern threatened to make a mockery of my commitment.

This time, however, I had a few things in my favor. One, celibacy had not been forced upon me. I had chosen it, indeed, welcomed it with open arms. Two, I was no longer young and inexperienced. Three, I had set for myself a goal of healing old hurts and becoming aware of destructive relationship patterns so that I would never repeat them again.

I began to see the underlying dynamics of our attraction for each other. Instead of viewing him as some godlike being, I began to see him as he was—a man, full of goodness and full of flaws. Inevitably, we found ourselves alone, which put me face-to-face with my celibacy promise. Did I mean to keep it or not? I wavered, but only for a moment. Technically I remained celibate, but what really helped me break the pattern of this relationship was that I remembered a vow I had made to myself long ago—that if our paths ever crossed again and sex became an issue, I would say no. My promise had been a vow, prayer, and fear all wrapped up into one. But as I remembered it and the painful circumstances that had produced those words, I received strength and a sense of determination that I had never before felt with him. *I would not have sex with this man.*

I'll admit, the first time we were alone together, it was difficult to say no. But somehow, from somewhere, I mustered the strength to tell this man no. He was surprised; in the past, I had always said yes. On another occasion, he tried to seduce me, but again I said no. He tried again and again, and amazingly, after a while, it became easy.

"No, I don't think so," I said sweetly.

"No no no!" I sang.

"Noooo!" I cried.

"Hell, no!" I said, snapping my fingers.

> ISAAC NEWTON, THE MATHEMATICIAN AND SCIENTIST (SAID BY SOME TO BE THE GREATEST SCIENTIST EVER), WAS A VIRGIN ALL HIS LIFE. HE WAS ALSO VERY UNPOPULAR.
> —THE CELIBATE FAQ

My practice of celibacy, wholeheartedly entered into and willingly committed to, was the tool my God used to clear my sight and calm my heart. I really wanted this man, but the more I said no to him, the stronger I felt in my position. Also, for the first time, I finally understood why we were not a good match, and rather than perpetuate a destructive pattern, I chose to annihilate it. I saved myself from what would undoubtedly have been yet another heartbreaking experience and a few more years of trying to heal. I felt that I'd passed a major test.

This experience confirmed for me the power inherent in a healthy celibacy practice. It was my change in attitude that made all the difference. I did not feel as if I was forced into celibacy—I chose to become celibate. I set goals, laid out a plan, and implemented various activities that brought about some wonderful manifestations. Best of all, I finally made peace with myself. Through an intense process of prayer, meditation, and self-reflection, I finally came to see the goodness that was inside me. I learned to like and love the person that I am. But first I had to honestly face those aspects of myself that I perceived made me unworthy, unlovable. Coming face-to-face with oneself is not easy. It's not fun. Sometimes it can be downright painful. But I can honestly and happily report that it's well worth the effort.

Testing the Waters

Since the moment you made your decision to practice celibacy, several months—maybe years—have gone by. Despite the opportunities for sex, you've stuck to your decision to practice celibacy for a time. You've gained some valuable self-knowledge and have begun to explore other bands of the play spectrum. You're even beginning to achieve some of your goals. Life may not be perfect (who ever promised us that?), but it is satisfying and at times even fun. And not once did you explode from sexual pressure!

Still, you can't shake the desire for love, romance, relationship, and marriage. You crave companionship and intimate friendship with a man. That's good. That means you're healing from bitterness, rage, and sorrow. You're ready to risk love again. I applaud you. A healthy celibacy practice seldom leads to "sexual anorexia" or monasticism but to a heightened appreciation, empathy, and desire for the opposite sex.

But can you trust yourself? you wonder. You've made such disastrous mistakes in the past with men, can you really trust yourself to make an intelligent decision this time? Going back out into the world is never a sure thing—that's why it's called a risk—but going back out there is the only way to address your soul's needs for loving companionship and hot sex with your soul mate. Trust yourself; trust in your ability to make this Program a positive, healing force in your life.

Can you trust men, though? That's the question. Your experiences with men in the past have probably been very painful. If only you didn't desire their companionship, life would be so much simpler. The reality is, we need them, and they need us. In the past, you might have gotten into relationships as half a person with no self-knowledge, self-worth, or self-love. More than likely, you resonated to men who had the same issues because like attracts like. Relationship math says that two halves do not make a whole, they make two halves. Today you're a new woman, more aware, wise, and healed. Thus you will be attracted to more emotionally mature men. One whole + one whole = one interdependent loving unit.

Jerks will still come and go, and you may even be attracted to one or two of them, but you'll begin to think twice before jumping into bed. Shortly before meeting Father #2, I met a man to whom I was wildly attracted. My feelings had no rhyme or reason, they just were. So we went out to dinner to decide what to do about all this sexual tension. Amazingly, I had the presence of mind to ask this man an important question: "Are you involved with anyone?" To his credit, he told me the truth: "Yes." Disappointed, I told him that I couldn't get involved. He wanted to know why. I told him about my policy of not getting mixed up with married or otherwise involved men. (I still hadn't learned to ask questions like "Do I know you? Are our goals for love, commitment, and marriage compatible? Do we have similar values, an 'equally yoked' spiritual approach to life? Are we really ready to take that step into the sack, or are we just responding to animal magnetism?" I would learn to ask these kinds of questions much later.)

At this point, the real man started to emerge. He couldn't understand why I was making such a fuss. After all, we were only talking about sex. To him, sex was just something two people do. To me, sex meant love and marriage (which is why I can't do it with just any old body). To him, sex was about making a deposit. To me, sex meant that I would receive his essence into my body and spirit. Interestingly, the more he talked, the less I liked him. With one question, I saved myself quite a bit of wear and tear because I'm sure that had I gone to bed with him, I would have had to fall in love with him and that would have gotten messy.

All types of men will parade through your life, but now that you're armed with self-knowledge, healing, and some life-mission goals, you should be attracted to a different kind of man. That does not mean that you'll be able to predict how a man will behave in the long run, nor will you be able to control his attitudes or behaviors. If your hidden agenda for your self-improvement program is to manipulate and dominate situations and people, you're on the wrong track and you are misusing the Program.

The truth is, you may have to date a couple of frogs before you settle down with the right man. *The Rules* and similar books that advocate behavioral change to hog-tie men may help prevent the "fatal attraction" approach to dating, but they can't guarantee a quality mate. Also, *The Rules* asks the questions: Do you really want a man that you have to manipulate? Shouldn't the goal be honesty and authenticity in relationships? If you begin a relationship dishonestly, you'll have to keep up the act, maybe for the rest of your life.

During the course of the Sensual Celibacy Program, you've been changing aspects of yourself that no longer serve you. As you start testing the dating waters again, this time as a woman practicing celibacy, your approach to dating and intimate relationships will have to change too. Game playing devalues men and women. Learning how to communicate clearly and honestly and having realistic expectations should be our goals.

With that in mind, I present to you the Sensual Celibacy Dating Bill of Rights and Responsibilities:

+ Every woman has the right to pursue love, liberty, and happiness.

+ Every woman has the right to say no to sex if she's not ready.

+ Every woman practicing celibacy must have the courage of her convictions.

+ Every woman must have a strong sense of her own boundaries.

+ Every woman must respect a man's decision to move on if he doesn't want to abstain from sex.

+ Every woman has the right to forgiveness if she falls off the wagon.

+ Every woman has the right to date as many men as she can manage.

+ Every woman has the duty to continue her self-improvement program whether or not she is in a relationship with a man.

Let's explore these rights and responsibilities in greater depth.

EVERY WOMAN HAS THE RIGHT TO PURSUE LOVE, LIBERTY, AND HAPPINESS. Why should couples have all the fun? Single women and men, whether in relationships or not, have the right to pursue healthy love relationships. This may seem obvious, but I often hear people, usually married, encouraging singles to be happy with their single state. Something about the grass always being greener on the other side.

This is nonsense. Married people wouldn't be married if they hadn't pursued love. To tell a single person to deny her soul's longings is irresponsible and makes me wonder about the real reasons behind such advice.

So pursue! Skip *The Rules!* Approach men that you find attractive. Think of it this way: You'd introduce yourself to another woman as a gesture of friendship or in the interest of career networking, wouldn't you? You wouldn't be afraid to call her up for coffee, would you? If you approach men with that same friendly attitude, you're going to be meeting and dating men in no time.

EVERY WOMAN HAS THE RIGHT TO SAY NO TO SEX IF SHE'S NOT READY. Once you start dating, it's a given: You will receive pressure to have sex. If you are not ready for sex, *you don't have to do it.*

Telling a man no doesn't have to be an uncomfortable moment if you lay the groundwork early on.

+ Tell your friend about your celibacy promise as soon as possible.

+ In the beginning stages of a relationship, do not let him in your apartment, and don't go to his. Meet in public places.

+ Old-style dieting is hard because you deny yourself all your favorite foods. Old-style celibacy is the same way. The woman practicing Sensual Celibacy is only saying no to one small band of the play spectrum or the intimacy spectrum. Although your answer to sex is no right now, you're saying yes to so many more things. So the next time a man wants to have sex with you before you are ready, say *yes* to wisdom, *yes* to your celibacy promise, *yes* to relationship commitment/marriage first, *yes* to life, *yes* to love, *yes* to deeper intimacy—but no to sex.

✦ *Isometric thigh squeeze:* Close your legs and squeeze your thighs tightly for as long as necessary. Great for toning the thighs and prevents penile penetration.

✦ Remember your sexual triggers. You now know some of the romantic situations that could make you "forget" your promise to yourself. Don't go goo-goo eyed and unconscious. The romantic feelings are wonderful, but that doesn't mean you go to sleep. Despite how you and millions of women in the past and present have done it, you don't have to deny your ability to reason through a romantic situation. In other words, don't lose your mind. Stay awake and aware. No woman working this Program has the right to say "sex just happened." That's a cop-out. You are now armed with information about yourself, and now you need time to get to know your new man. You can't effectively do that if you're accidentally having sex.

✦ Take responsibility, not unnecessary chances, especially if you're with someone new. Don't party too hard. Women who are under the influence of drugs or alcohol often don't get the chance to say no or can't make their positions clear. Their right to decide can be stolen from them. Beware.

When you just say no, make sure that no really means no. If you're not firm in your resolve, any bad boy will be able to detect your uncertainty. He'll assume that your no really means yes and that you're just playing coy and hard to get. This may be the green light he needs to pursue you full thrust. If you're not firm in your resolve, a virtuoso will play your sexual triggers like the strings on a violin. At first his attention and ardor may be flattering, but in the end you may be the one to suffer.

EVERY WOMAN PRACTICING CELIBACY MUST HAVE THE COURAGE OF HER CONVICTIONS. You may experience ridicule for your decision to practice celibacy. During the days when celibacy and virginity were the norm, sexually active women were called "whores" and "sluts." The tables have turned, and we women practicing celibacy sometimes find ourselves the subjects of jokes and finger-pointing. Maybe one day we will all grow up and learn to appreciate and respect diversity of lifestyles and viewpoints, but until that day, you can not let the words of others harm you or deter you from the promise you made to yourself. You made the decision to practice celibacy as an act of self-love, and it was a good decision. Stand on that.

EVERY WOMAN MUST HAVE A STRONG SENSE OF HER OWN BOUNDARIES. Remember your celibacy type from chapter 4? If you're a Ten Commandments Celibate, then you know that sex and probably heavy petting are off-limits until marriage. If you're a Moderate Celibate, you won't be ready to have sex until you feel reasonably sure that you're in a committed, monogamous, healthy, loving relationship.

Technical Celibates are some of my favorite people. "Can't I have just a little bit?" is their approach to dating. However, even these earthy, passionate women must have a strong sense of just how far they can go on a date. It is for them that I offer the following Passionmeter:

talking → holding hands → eye gazing → sweet talk → kissing → tongue kissing → grinding → clothes coming off → clothes off → doing the deed

Each one of the steps to sex on the meter contains an opportunity to stop—except, of course, the last one. The further to the right you go, the harder it will be to stop. You know you've entered into the land of no return when the penis has penetrated. You've fallen off the wagon.

I also worry about the safety of some Technical Celibates. Declaring sex off-limits but picking up men the way Diane Keaton did in *Looking for Mr. Goodbar* is dangerous, foolhardy, and may indicate a sexual addiction. Get counseling—your life may depend on it.

"Know thyself" should be the motto of any woman who is dating, whether she is celibate or not. Know your sexual triggers. Know why you're involved with a man. No longer can you say, "I don't know what happened. We were kissing, and the next thing you know—" No more accidental sex. Review your list of sexual triggers regularly. The goal is to keep them in your conscious level of awareness. Don't go to sleep on them because that's when they'll work most powerfully on you. Finally, make a concerted effort to incorporate the solo conversions you created in chapter 7 into your life. The more you treat yourself to sensuality on a day-by-day, moment-to-moment basis, the less you'll feel deprived and vulnerable to seduction before you're ready.

EVERY WOMAN MUST RESPECT A MAN'S DECISION TO MOVE ON IF HE DOESN'T WANT TO ABSTAIN FROM SEX. Just because you have decided to practice celibacy doesn't mean that your dates have. In fact, you may find that your budding relationships quickly turn platonic, or even hostile, once you've announced your "no sex" stand. A man never has a right to emotionally, physically, or verbally abuse you out of anger because of your declaration, but he does have the right to walk away.

How you tell a man about your decision is as important as *what* you tell him. I recommend saying something simple like "I just thought you should know that I'm practicing celibacy during this time of my life." Carefully monitor yourself for any feelings of self-righteousness, superiority, or shame, because how you feel will be communicated to your date. Nor should you try and sell your date on celibacy. If he's curious about your decision, then by all means tell him as much as you feel comfortable disclosing. Some men will hear you out, others won't have the slightest interest. Mostly, talk about your interests—that's much bigger than your practice of celibacy.

A couple of years ago, my friend Frances met a man, liked him, and agreed to go out with him. The first date went smoothly, so they scheduled a second date. While they were driving to the restaurant, he played an audiocassette tape of a minister talking to an audience of young people about the benefits of staying virgins until marriage. His playing the tape made Frances feel comfortable about her celibacy decision, which she'd explained on their first date.

After dinner, they went up to his apartment. Big mistake, but Frances thought her decision was going to be respected. The next thing she knew, she was frantically pushing the man off her. He had gone so far as to un-snap her bra. Fortunately, he got the message and let her go. Frightened out of her mind, she got out of his apartment as fast as she could. Date rape is no joke, so don't put yourself in a compromising situation. Frances was very lucky. No means no, but some men won't respect your bound-aries because they have none of their own. A man's apartment should be off-limits until you really get to know him, and that takes time.

Ideally, your disclosure of your practice will help you weed out the bad boys from the good.

EVERY WOMAN HAS THE RIGHT TO FORGIVENESS IF SHE FALLS OFF THE WAGON. A couple of years ago I fell off the wagon. No, I jumped off. Having sex with a man that you care about and love is not a bad thing to do. Sex is a normal and natural expression of love and attraction. Without a commitment, however, the relationship will get messy if sex is involved.

This man was a repeat, i.e., we had had a relationship several years before. It had ended vaguely back then, and the lack of closure left me with many unanswered questions. I still had feelings for him, so, more or less, we picked up where we had left off.

Now I'm clear. It only took a few short months to find out that the emotionally unavailable man I knew many years ago was still wounded and unavailable. Once I got the closure I needed, I easily climbed back on the wagon. The knowledge I gained during the encounter was something I needed in order to move forward.

Being a sex sym-bol was rather like being a convict.

—RAQUEL WELCH

Some may think I am a failure because I jumped off the wagon, but I don't see it that way. Since I try not to attach any religious dogma to my practice of celibacy, I don't feel that I sinned or that I'm going to hell for loving a man. That does not mean there's no price to pay. For every decision you make or don't make in life, there are consequences. However, I am free to analyze and inter-pret the events in my life as I feel led by that silent, inner Voice, which is a blessing. Having that relationship was necessary to close a chapter in my life. In no way did that involvement diminish the success of my celibacy practice. It was because of the progress I made up to that point that I was able to decisively and quickly end the relationship. In only a short few months, I understood that this was not for me, and I cut the strings with no regrets. Without a strong celibacy practice prior to the relationship, I might have allowed it to go on much too long. I learned and grew from the experience. I forgave us both and went on with my life.

EVERY WOMAN HAS THE RIGHT TO DATE AS MANY MEN AS SHE CAN MANAGE. Debrena Jackson Gandy, author of *Sacred Pampering Principles,* recommends that a woman date three men at a time until she settles into one monogamous commitment. "It takes a truly magical woman to keep three men interested without any sexual involvement." Three is a good number, but if you can handle more, go for it. Until you are ready to commit to one man, date as many men as your time, energy, and resources will allow.

Make friends with men. Get to know them first as human beings. Demystify them. Practice being yourself around men. Listen to them, but also learn to share your own hopes, dreams, and desires. Don't lapse into the *Rules* trap by hiding your unique sparkle under fake smiles and reserve. Be authentic, be real.

EVERY WOMAN HAS THE DUTY TO CONTINUE HER SELF-IMPROVEMENT PROGRAM WHETHER OR NOT SHE IS IN A RELATIONSHIP WITH A MAN. Don't ever lose yourself in a man. Continue to pursue your dreams. Your man was attracted to you because of your self-improvement efforts and your progress. Don't let the good feelings obscure your vision. Keep moving forward.

Approach dating with a playful attitude and, I reiterate, don't have sex before you're ready. There's a soul mate a'coming, and wouldn't it be a shame if you were busy with some other man just as your love paths crossed. Better to stay free and clear of all commitments until you're sure that *he's the one.*

MATING SEASON EXERCISE. Let's face it, if you're a healthy, sensuous woman, there will be times when all you want to do is have sex. Heaven help the celibate woman whose hormones are screaming, Have sex right now! Cuddling? Not today!

Mating season is different from your usual monthly sexual peaks and valleys. Mating season is that time of year when *you must have sex.* Your juices are flowing constantly, and all men, no matter how short or tall, fat or skinny, rich or poor, look mighty tasty. Mating season's the time to get down. Recently I was telling a friend that springtime is my mating season and that both of my children were conceived just as the buds on the red maples were peeking through. My friend threatened to put me under lock and key until winter.

Complicating mating season is your celibacy practice. If you're in a monogamous, committed, healthy, loving relationship with a man, all's right with the world, and mating season is a good time. But if you' re celibate, you will have to call on all your strength of will and all your sensual celibacy skills to not do something you'll inevitably regret. If you're not already involved with a man, it's best to not get involved with anyone at this time because your lower regions are doing all the thinking for you.

In his work with Australian Aborigines, author and artist Robert Lawlor found that many tribes believe that to ensure the peace of a community, the sexual appetites of all mature women must be satisfied, regardless of whether they are nineteen or ninety. They believe that sexually inactive women create chaos and turmoil within the tribe. Says Lawlor in his book *Voices of the First Day: Awakening in the Aboriginal Dreamtime,* "A sexually dissatisfied wife may, if unable to find an extra-marital liaison, generate unimaginable domestic disharmony." At all costs, women must be kept sexually satisfied.

Ladies, think about it: When you want to have sex, and none is available, what do you feel (besides horny)? Frustration. Irritation. Rage. Depression. If Shere Hite is correct and *at least* one-third of American women are not having sex, what does this do to our emotional health? To our group consciousness? If I were a researcher, I'd like to know how celibacy (the neurotic kind usually practiced in this country) impacts the Nielsen ratings and the gross national product!

During mating season, celibate women are at risk of depression. It's easy to forget that celibacy does not have to mean grimness and bondage, because it can sure feel that way. Just remember, though, that celibacy does not have to mean lack of love and sensuality. If your wild woman is caged, you will die a slow, painful death. You can actually get sick. But if you let her out and play, you'll be able to tolerate the discipline of celibacy even under the most trying hormonal and seasonal conditions.

How to handle this season, still keep your sanity, and not fall off the wagon?

+ *Let your wild woman out!* Do something physical and fun. Dance to some funky music and shake those hips. Ride a horse. Take deep deep breaths, and take them often. Take a belly dancing class. When you do exercises such as the pelvic tilt, let your imagination run wild. Go to the park and swing. Ride a roller coaster. When you walk, switch your hips more deliberately. If you try and beat your sexuality into submission, this powerful life force may erupt in ways that are not healthy. Better to go with the flow. Learn to enjoy the feelings without having to have sex. It can be done.

+ *Hug at least ten people every day.* Everyone needs to be touched and held. Babies wither and die if they don't receive regular doses of loving tactile stimulation. You may have learned how to cope, but the truth is, you need to be touched just as much as babies do. Hold hands with a child. Hold your pet. Go to temple/mosque/synagogue/church: There are plenty of hugs to go around. Get a massage. Get your hugs and touches today!

+ *Breathe in male energy.* Go to a place where lots of men gather (sporting events, billiards clubs). Flirt with them, be around them—just don't go home with them. Sometimes all you need is some attention. If you' re approached by a man and you're interested, keep him dangling for another season or so. There's no way you'll be able to make a rational decision right now. If he's still around by winter, and you're still interested, it might be love.

✦ *Be kind to yourself.* Because depression is such an ever-present threat during mating season, it is more important than ever to be kind to yourself. Do not berate yourself for having normal, healthy womanly feelings. Pamper yourself. If you can afford it, get a massage, buy yourself a new outfit, take a trip, redecorate your bedroom in sensuous colors. If you're on a budget, take the time to groom yourself in bold new ways. Pluck your eyebrows, give yourself a pedicure and paint your toes red (to match the fire *down there*), hem up a skirt to let your beautiful knees show. Eat well; prepare dishes from only the freshest foods, herbs, and spices. Most important, give yourself permission to feel down occasionally. After all, practicing celibacy during mating season goes against the call of nature. You're supposed to be doing it to some delicious hunk of a man. Don't feel bad about feeling bad, just try not to wallow in the depression. Face it with courage and get into prayer and meditation. Trust that your body, mind, and heart will be sustained during this challenging time. You will not blow up from the sexual pressure!

AFFIRMATION: *I am strong and can keep my celibacy promise to myself even when I don't want to. I will have sex when I'm ready and not a moment before.*

CHAPTER TEN

Step 8—
Give Men the Benefit
of the Doubt

Can you love a virgin man?

—Smokey Robinson

✦ ✦ ✦

Are there men out there who will honor your commitment to celibacy? Hard to imagine, but yes, there are. It just takes some looking, patience, and a willingness to educate the men with whom you come in contact.

The idea of the red-blooded American Joe understanding, sympathizing with, and agreeing to practice celibacy is a stretch for many of our imaginations, but before we judge all men as close-minded clods, let's give them the benefit of the doubt. Let's not just automatically assume that your men will run away. Some will, but not all.

There are four basic types of men when it comes to responding to your celibacy practice:

1. *The See Ya Man.* The moment you say no to sex is the moment he excuses himself from the table and bolts for the door. This man is frankly interested in sexual relationships, and that's his prerogative. Just be thankful that he had the decency to leave right away.

2. *Casanova.* Tell this man no to sex, and suddenly, you're the object of his most ardent attentions. You'll receive flowers, cards, and daily calls. If he's rich you might even get a blue box from Tiffany's. This guy's a real charmer, and if you don't keep your wits about you, you could fall hard. Casanovas are masters at identifying and playing women's sexual triggers. This is the one area in which they excel because they've made the conquest of women a lifelong career. Remember, you're a challenge, and he wants to conquer you. Once he's succeeded, he'll be on the heels of the See Ya Man. How to identify a Casanova? Keep saying no. Talk to him. Get him to talk about his past. If he keeps shifting the conversation to you, if he seems reluctant to talk about himself, you might have a problem on your hands. Just keep saying no. Refer back to the resistance strategies in the last chapter. Trust your gut. If the guy seems too good to be true, he probably is.

3. *The Scholar.* Now here's a man worth considering. The Scholar has never seriously thought about celibacy in the past because he never had to. But now that you've brought it up, he's intrigued. And if he's interested in you, he could be convinced to share your celibacy experience. He may not mind taking your lead because, more or less, he's secure in his masculinity. He's open to being educated. Don't mistake his probing questions for rejection. That he is talking to you about celibacy at all says a lot about his open-mindedness and his feelings for you. If he finally decides that he cares about you enough to give celibacy a try, he may not feel comfortable talking about it to his friends. He may want to stay in the closet. Don't hold it against him. The most important thing is that he's respecting your decision. Don't be surprised, however, if he tries, from time to time, to get you to change your mind. Stand firm until you are ready to have sex with him.

4. *The Renaissance Man.* This man is a rare and precious jewel. The Renaissance Man is already a believer in, and maybe even a practitioner of, celibacy. There aren't many of him around, but this type of man does exist. I even talked to a couple of them for this chapter. They have strongly held convictions about honoring their bodies and the women they become involved in. One man I spoke to was a committed Ten Commandments Celibate. As you become stronger in your convictions about your celibacy practice, you'll be amazed at the quality of people who will cross your path. Don't be surprised if you begin to meet Renaissance Men. If you have the good fortune to become romantically involved with one, you start out with trust on certain issues, like fidelity. This guy is big on friendship and getting to know each other first, rather than trying to achieve instant intimacy through sex—and that's refreshing. In the past, "getting to first base" was about a man's attempt to have sex with you. The Renaissance Man redefines getting to first base as an attempt to have an honest meeting of the minds and heart.

Of course, get to know him first, but you can trust him to

not hang out with the Casanova crowd. The shadow side of the Renaissance Man is that he may be hard to get close to. He may be judgmental and intolerant of your sexual history. He may or may not be practicing a self-loving approach to celibacy, in which case you might want to run. If he is celibate because of religious reasons, then his practice may be colored by a lot of dogma. You'll have to decide whether you can handle that or not. If you really like this man, however, give him a chance.

For many women, male celibacy feels like a personal rejection. I too have had mixed feelings about male celibacy. We have all been so brainwashed to think that men must have sex all the time that when we actually meet a man who respects his body and self enough to say no to casual sex, we wonder what's wrong with him. Yet we women have decided to abstain from casual sex; shouldn't we be seeking out, making friends with, and giving our full support to our kindred brothers?

There's a fifty-fifty chance that your man might consider practicing celibacy with you—if he's really interested in you. The timing has to be right for both of you.

The purpose of this chapter is to clear up some of the misconceptions and myths about male celibacy and male sexuality. In addition:

+ Today, the traditional male image, behaviors, and attitudes are being challenged, and many men are feeling confused and threatened. They're trying to find their way just like we are. Since much of their identity revolves around sexuality and virility, your celibacy may very well pose a tremendous threat.

+ Some men, not many, but some, are turning to celibacy as a viable alternative to casual sex. Some of their issues and reasons for abstinence may differ from ours, and they warrant a closer look.

What Is a Real Man?

Does the phrase "celibate man" sound like an oxymoron to you? Can you even form your lips to say the words "celibate" and "man" together?

What image does the term "celibate man" conjure in your mind? A man dressed in priestly robes and a white collar? An ancient-looking man, hunched over, with no life left in him? Can you imagine a celibate man as a young, healthy, good-looking man between the ages of twenty and forty-five? Could you imagine Denzel Washington and Tom Cruise as celibate men? Would you *want* to imagine them as celibate?

If the Hollywood spin machine can't afford to let an adoring public think of their favorite male stars as gay, they certainly can't afford to let us in on their celibacy secrets. In our society, celibacy is perceived as the great emasculator of men. Forget the tremendous discipline, courage, and strength of will that men must draw upon to keep their celibacy promise. The idea of male celibacy destroys our fantasy of the masculine mystique, that virile, handsome, sexual charmer who is the object of our wildest fantasies.

The very definition of manhood includes the aspect of sexual vigor—or, at the very least, sexual involvement. A man must be having sex with somebody to be a card-carrying man in this United States of America. If a man is not sexually involved, he'd better be on the prowl, lest his reputation suffer the disapproval of male peers, females, and so-ciety. And that's how we raise our boys. Right away they learn that in order to hold their heads up high, they must "score" (always playing) and quick.

Prior to researching and writing this book, the phrase "celibate man" was, for me, an oxymoron, like "dry rain" or "sensual celibacy." Putting those two words together had the same effect on my brain cells as bells clanging, bombs dropping, and worlds colliding. I knew of no such exotic species of human as a man who did not have sex. Every man I had ever known was having sex, and lots of it.

Or so I thought.

Ladies, we've all been sold a bill of goods. We are well aware of the strange compulsion of teenage boys to claim sexual experience before they've even seen a girl's upper thigh. Why should we think grown boys, i.e., *men*, are any different? All the claims of sexual "hits" to the contrary, men have their vacation times just like we do. The difference is, it is more acceptable for women to talk about it. Unfortunately, men usually keep their practice of celibacy a deep, dark secret that has the power to shame and disgrace them if revealed.

On a sheet of paper, list all the men, past and present, who you personally knew were practicing celibacy. Now exclude from your list all sick and dying men. Exclude all young men under the age of twenty. Exclude all Professional Celibates, e.g., monks and priests. Exclude all impotent men. As your list gets smaller and smaller (if you had any names listed at all), you'll probably begin to realize that you don't know many, if any, men who are practicing celibacy.

Yet you probably know more sexually abstaining men than you realize. Many men find admitting the truth about the absence of sex in their lives more difficult than expressing emotions. In fact, men will go out of their way to make up and tell sexual conquest stories to anyone who will listen.

To understand why men feel the need to lie about their celibacy, we must explore men's tendency to lie about everything. Just kidding. Seriously, we women explain away some of the most confusing male behavior with one sweeping explanation: men are simple. When men lie, they're being simple. When they cheat, they're being simple. We compare men to dogs in perpetual heat. Dogs are simple—give them a pretty pooch and some chow and they're happy. Give a real man the same, however, and he's restless for more and feeling empty inside. This is not simple dog instinct or behavior.

> *IF A FELLOW CEASES DATING YOU BECAUSE YOU REFUSE TO ENGAGE IN THE SEXUAL ACT, YOU CAN BE ASSURED THAT HE IS NOT GENUINELY INTERESTED IN YOU AND THEREFORE WOULD MAKE AN UNDESIRABLE HUSBAND.*
>
> —MARTIN LUTHER KING, JR.

Men as a group are much too complicated for us to reduce their bewildering behaviors to such explanations as "men lie" or "boys will be boys." Still, the myth of the simple male, otherwise known as a "guy," persists. Garrison Keillor and others have popularized the myth of the guy. Men may be straightforward, but they're not simple, not in the least. Men made the atom bomb. It was a man who discovered $E=mc^2$. Men run governments and multinational corporations. They make war and love with the same ferocity and passion. The same men who can drop bombs on entire nations can cry at the sight of a newborn baby or at the funeral of a loved one. Molly Katzen, author of the *Moosewood Cookbook,* says that her father cried real tears at the first taste of a Jewish dish his wife served him.

This is not amoeba behavior here, and we underestimate men by reducing them to simple liars, cheats, and incompetents. So if they're so smart, how come they fail time and again to give us women what we need? you may ask. I never said they were smart; I said they were complex. Given our behavior with them, I can't say we're any smarter. We're both in the same boat. Since we know little about what makes the other tick, neither side has a healthy appreciation for the uniqueness of the other. Furthermore, our ignorance is driving us both crazy.

Volumes have been written about the female psyche, and if men would take the time to study and talk to us openly and honestly, they'd learn a thing or two. Likewise, if we women would, as the book says, begin to open our hearts and minds to men, we'd learn a thing or two.

One of the greatest stumbling blocks men have to overcome in order to become healthy, happy human beings is their mass denial of emotions. Men have emotions, but they don't deal with them effectively. Women's insistence on analyzing every shade and nuance of a feeling drives men insane. They just want to get to the solution part of the dispute and go on to something, anything else. Many men look down their noses at women's many intelligences, so few of them have taken the time to develop the so-called feminine faculties, such as intuition, sensuality, and emotion. In the realm of male emotions, only two are socially allowed: anger/rage and lust.

Herein lies our confusion: Men say one thing, but usually mean and feel something else. That's not simple behavior. Our cynicism and distrust prevent us from understanding the true nature of men. Our desire and desperation for men blinds us to their true intentions. Men often say that women don't want to know the truth, that we just want the fantasy. So they give us what they think we want to get what they think they want. The result is a big mess.

I have been seduced by the words "I love you" (hearing this phrase is a sexual trigger for most women) more times than I care to admit. A man will say those three words with intensity, urgency, and complete believability, so we wonder, How could he leave? How could he do or say such a thing? Most men will admit to having uttered these three words at least once to get sex. It's an unhealthy deal that serves our temporary needs while undermining our long-term ones: The man gets his sex, and the woman gets her fantasy. Truth has not been served in either case.

I've come to another conclusion, though this one may be perceived as somewhat controversial. Based on my experience and the hundreds of conversations I have had with men and women on this issue over the past few years, I have come to the conclusion that when a man says "I love you," he really means it. We women rant and rave about men being liars and dogs, but to be truly guilty of some of the attitudes and behaviors laid upon them, men, as a group, would have to be theologically judged as Satan incarnate; clinically diagnosed as sociopaths or at the very least sexual addicts; or judiciously labeled as criminals.

How dare I say that men really mean it when they say they love you? No doubt every woman in the world has a story to tell about having been abandoned, cheated on, and lied to, but before you shut the book in disgust, let me quickly clarify: *At the moment* a man is professing his undying love, he really means it. When women say "I love you," we have begun the bonding process. Our minds are racing to the altar, and our hearts have made a quantum leap into "intimacy." We want to spend more time with our beloved. We want to pick out silverware patterns together, make a life together. When men say "I love you," they stay a minute, establish their home base through lovemaking and pillow talk, then move on to the next adventure, be it work or hanging out with the fellas (or another woman). A minute in man-time equals a couple of months in woman-time, but it only takes a moment for the entire relationship to blow up.

At the risk of appearing to justify the shadow side of male behavior, I sometimes think that women's anger at men subconsciously stems from men's resistance to being domesticated. Are we jealous of men's ability to roam the globe without having to worry about staying put long enough to birth, feed, clothe, and educate babies? I know fathers who seldom ever talk to their children, and I don't know how they do it. I think about women like Coretta Scott King and Jackie Kennedy Onassis, the women "behind" Martin Luther King, Jr., and John F. Kennedy, respectively. While their husbands were out in the limelight, these women seemed content to stay behind and take care of hearth and home. Or were they?

It is a rare man who can accept his domestication with grace, humor, and style. The women I know who are married to such gems usually get restless and bored *because* their men are domesticated. Go figure. These women bemoan the fact that their husbands work, come home, take care of the kids, and watch TV. I guess they want to go out disco dancing or something. Now if their men were out roaming the streets, they'd be crying. There's just no pleasing some women. To them I say this: Go live for a day in the shoes of a single woman who has no one, save her cats and maybe a child or two, to share the joys and trials of her life with her. Then run back home and do something special for your husband. *Be grateful* for him. He is rare.

Many men say that they want a good woman, but their own unresolved issues keep them running. In our society, therapy is emasculating (a real man handles his business), so many continue self-destructive patterns of pursuit, conquest, and flight until they die. And marriage is no guarantee that the pattern will end.

Why do men act this way? What exotic gene do men have? After my many years of in-the-trenches research, I've finally learned the secrets to understanding what makes men act the way they do:

+ Men have short attention spans for women.

+ Men have long attention spans for play.

That's not to say that playful men are irresponsible or bad. Many admirably fulfill their obligations as fathers, adult sons, entrepreneurs, employees, etc. But ask them what turns them on besides sex, and most often their answers will have little to do with the woman they love most in life. They'll talk about their love of sports, their work, music, hobbies, and their buddies.

There are so many books on the market for women that focus on using sex as a trap to snare male prey—how to satisfy a man in bed, how to drive a man wild, how to turn a man on and on. Don't get me wrong, sex is extremely important to men, but by focusing on sex, we women do ourselves a disservice by compartmentalizing ourselves out of the other areas of a man's life. To understand a man is to know his play passions. Men have had the freedom to tap into and regularly enjoy realms of existence other than sex. They are so good at playing that they can even turn work and war into games. During sex, we women only get to see one side of a man, and they only get to see one side of us. One of the benefits of celibacy is that it offers both genders opportunities to explore the other bands of the play spectrum together. Once intimacy has been achieved in this way, sex is much more explosive and fun. Best of all, there is more balance in the relationship. Women are no longer relegated to the periphery of men's lives.

The Men's Movement

What is Man? That very question lies at the heart of the men's movement today. In the '60s, women asked, What is Woman? and the culture changed overnight. Likewise, as men embark on that journey popularly known as "consciousness-raising," the culture will continue to evolve.

The men's movement is exciting. When men get together to heal, you have to sit up and take notice. We women have laughed at the idea of men gathering together out in the woods to beat their drums and chests. We fear a return to male dominance from the thousands of Christian men who participate in Promise Keepers conventions. We were angry that one million African-American men prohibited our participation on the Day of Atonement. But we shouldn't feel threatened. We should feel hopeful that the best in men that has been hidden all along will begin to emerge as they regroup among themselves.

The men's movement appears to be a full frontal attack against macho, bravado, cool, and posturing. We can only hope. Men are talking about dealing with emotions, arguably their biggest challenge. At last they are acknowledging the little boy inside who still smarts at the memory of how neither father nor society allowed emotion, creativity, or gentleness. It's the child who holds the keys to the inner kingdom.

What freedom it is to be able to say "I am afraid." For a man to admit fear, however, is to fail the manhood test. Men who admit fear are called "less than a man" and "punk." We never let our boys be afraid. They are initiated into pseudo-manhood via fighting, peer dares, and more, and heaven help them if they waver for a moment. Fear is a part of our emotional repertoire for a reason: Fear gives us a healthy respect for fires and nuclear bombs, among other things. As men emerge into the fullness of their manhood, they must acknowledge and come to grips with their fears.

One of men's biggest fears is that they won't perform well sexually. Most men will brag about their ability to please a woman. After the act (before he falls asleep), he'll usually ask, "Was it good for you, baby?" He asks because he truly doesn't know. A man once told my sister that he blanks out mentally during sex. Why? Because he's always afraid that he's not pleasing his partner. We might think "was it good for you?" is a leading question designed to elicit ego-stroking, but in truth, men are often extremely insecure about their sexual skills, energy levels, penis size, masculine image, etc.

Another big fear that men have is that they'll be caught practicing celibacy. One man who agreed to be interviewed for this chapter, under promise of anonymity, reneged at the last minute. He didn't want to risk anyone finding out that he hadn't had sex for a year and one-half.

Men are afraid of being caught with their pants up for the following reasons:

Constant sexual involvement defines the American version of manhood. According to this widely held belief, if you're not having sex, you're not a man. You're not even a boy. You're a "punk," a "wimp," and "gay." (The latter is the most ludicrous of all; I don't know one gay man who practices celibacy.)

A man who practices celibacy has psychological or physical problems. According to some schools of thought, there may be a fear of intimacy, low sex drive, shyness, or physical problems.

One celibate man I interviewed said that he definitely wanted a relationship that included sex, but that he valued his body too much to just have sex with any old body; thus, he was willing to wait. When I met him, he'd been celibate for a little more than a year. Another man I talked to had been celibate for most of the past seven years. He too wanted an intimate relationship but not outside of marriage. As a younger man, he was not ready for marriage. Now, in his mid-thirties, he is ready and is searching for his Ms. Right.

These two men do not have a lack of sexual interest nor are they any more afraid of an emotional involvement than the rest of us. They had both been in long-term relationships before. Sex therapists and authors who write on the subject of men and sex oversimplify the issues of celibacy, if they address it at all, and narrowly view male celibacy as an aberration.

In the Introduction, I talked about the dearth of research on celibacy. It's practically nonexistent for men. To find any information remotely connected to celibacy, you have to look up topic headings like "lack of interest" or "impotence." Yet men do practice celibacy from time to time; it's the most shameful secret of them all.

Men are not the only defenders of the order. Women are notorious for refusing to acknowledge and respect a man's decision to practice celibacy for a time. David, a friend of mine, told me that recently he was invited to spend an evening watching videos at the home of a female friend. She knew about his position on premarital sex. When he got to her apartment, guess where the TV was located? That's right, in the bedroom. The woman used all her wiles to try and get him to bed her, but he stood firm. "Are you gay?" she asked. "What's wrong with you?" Classic rejection responses.

David says those are the two questions women most frequently ask of him. When a woman is practicing celibacy, is she automatically asked, "Are you a lesbian?" There are double standards here, and we need to be aware of them as we meet more and more men on the path. Just as women have the right to say no, so do men. They deserve our kinship and support.

Celibacy is perceived as emasculating. "If you don't use it, you'll lose it" is the male credo. Celibacy is the complete antithesis to society's unforgiving and high expectations of male sexuality, and it takes courage and a strong sense of inner security for a man to abstain.

Vincent was the quintessential "man's man." If he was a woman, he would be called a whore or a slut. To say the least, he enjoyed a very busy sexual lifestyle.

Then came Suzanne. A Ten Commandments Celibate, she was firmly committed to her ideal of no premarital sex. Amazingly, Vincent agreed to her terms. Not only that, he never once cheated on her. For many years, I had my doubts about men's ability to delay instant sexual gratification, but after talking to Vincent and other men who have practiced or are practicing celibacy, my hope in men has been renewed. That's why this step in the Sensual Celibacy Program is an important one. If we give men the benefit of the doubt, if we give them a chance rather than jumping to negative conclusions about how they'll take to our celibacy practice, they might surprise us. Through celibacy we can develop some great relationships with men. The battle between the sexes could become a thing of the past!

The biological reality. One of the slogans for G. Heileman Ex-Imported Beer states, "Men think about Ex 100 times a day." Could Ex really be sex? Of course it is. Some studies have even gone so far as to document the number of times men think about sex in a day. One study found that men thought about sex more than 200 times a day.

Men are not animals, however. The instinct and drive to procreate are strong, but a man's mind is stronger. Much of what passes for biological drive is really a product of conditioning. The media incessantly reinforce the ideas that men are animals and that women are the sexual objects for which men lust.

Because masculinity is intertwined with sexuality, celibate men often dip in and out of experiences that help them maintain a tie, even an imaginary one, to their sexuality. Remember Michael Jackson's song "Beat It" and the accompanying video? Subliminal advertising expert Wilson Bryan Key saw a group male masturbation scene in the choreography (the way Michael was jerking and shaking his hand did look suspicious). Masturbation is a big issue with men in general, celibate men in particular. I had a friend who, married and forced into celibacy, was masturbating all day, every day. I was amazed to learn that men had that much sperm to release! While it helps a man keep his tie to his sexuality, excessive masturbation can make a frustrating situation worse.

I DON'T EVEN MASTURBATE ANYMORE, I'M SO AFRAID I'LL GIVE MYSELF SOMETHING. I JUST WANT TO BE FRIENDS WITH MYSELF.
—RICHARD LEWIS

Pornography also connects a man to his sexuality, albeit the low end. I used to work at a "high end" men's girlie magazine (no, not as a model), and I eventually quit because all those objectified breasts and pubic hairs were getting on my nerves. I regret that I, in my own small way, contributed to the delinquency (and shame) of many men and boys.

Masturbation and pornography work hand in glove, so to speak, but the underlying force that motivates men to seek out more sexual thrills is lust. Even Jimmy Carter had lust in his heart for a woman. Nature and nurture conspire to condition men to respond to women sexually, rather than as human beings. In the context of a marriage, or at least a loving, healthy, committed, monogamous relationship, a man's sexual desire for a woman is appropriate and beautiful. Desire outside that context becomes lust. It is just as problematic for a woman to want to be lusted after as a man who lusts in his heart. Lust requires an objectification of body parts and sexual organs. An individual's heart, mind, and soul are irrelevant.

If a man decides to deal with your celibacy, he's going to have to redefine manhood for himself, because he will quickly discover that the generally accepted social definition conflicts with a celibate lifestyle. He must learn to rely on other aspects of his character, values, and behaviors to touch the heart and essence of his manhood. For a man to grow into the fullness of his manhood while practicing celibacy, he must deal with self-doubt, fears, and occasional bouts of discouragement.

The Sensually Celibate Relationship

If your man says yes to the lifestyle, congratulations, you've found a treasure who just might go the distance. Living life as a celibate couple has its own rewards and its own challenges. Friendship can blossom beautifully in a relationship in which sex has been momentarily tabled. Friendship without sex provides a strong foundation for the soul mate aspect of the relationship. Instead of just focusing on erotic feelings, the two of you can explore other aspects of your lives and selves. When difficulties arise, you won't have sex to distract you.

Remember how we used to sit by the phone waiting for a man to call? Well, if your man keeps calling, despite not having sex with you, he may be interested.

For men and women sex produces much anxiety. Performance and body image are only two of the major fears. Sensual celibacy can calm those fears. In fact, this is the perfect opportunity to talk about such things. Without sex in your faces, you may not feel as threatened to talk about your sex-related fears.

Beware the Casanova, however. If your man only wants to talk about your sexual fantasies, your turn-ons, your sexual skills, then you might have a Casanova in disguise. If nine times out of ten your conversations end up being sexual, watch out. This man may just be agreeing to be celibate with you in order to get to your precious jewels. Beware. Casanovas are clever.

Once I dated a man for a few months who, on a daily basis, begged me for sex. When I told him right at the beginning that I was practicing celibacy, he asked with wide, innocent eyes, "Celibacy? What's that?" When he finally got it that I wasn't ready for sex, he'd complain, "You're making me sit over here like a eunuch." He tried having phone sex with me, and I'd tell him, "I'm not having phone sex with you." Once we were in his car and he tried to deepen the hug, so to speak. I firmly told him that I was not interested in car sex either. He'd start whining and begging so comically that I couldn't help but laugh. He claimed that he was making life so miserable for his coworkers that they were begging me to please "give him some."

*O*N THIS TRIP MY BED IS AS EMPTY AS YOURS, EXCEPT THAT MINE IS EMPTY BY CHOICE!

—CHIEF SCIENCE OFFI-CER DAX TO A KLINGON WARRIOR, *STAR TREK: DEEP SPACE NINE*

The more I said no to sex, the more he wanted it. He was a classic Casanova, a charmer. Thank God for celibacy, which gave me the emotional distance I needed to assess his true character.

If you and your man are practicing celibacy for a term, I guarantee there will be an ever-present desire for sex. We always want what we can't have. Your man sure does look good, and you want to be near him, and he wants you too. As love deepens, so does the desire for physical intimacy. This is good and normal. Some couples solve the dilemma by getting married (which may or may not be a good idea). Some just go ahead and accidentally have sex.

Down the road if your man starts to get frustrated with the whole idea and starts pressuring you to have sex, really consider whether you're ready or not. Or *you* may be feeling like this is it and let's go. Search your soul. Don't just go on automatic like you've done in the past. If you've been working this Program, you know too much about yourself now to go on automatic anyway. Get your journal out. Reread everything you've written about your sexual triggers, your ideas about men, sex, love, and relationships, and give it some hard thought. Some women might need time and space away from their heartthrob to think clearly. Take the time that you need, but understand that if his commitment to you is not all that deep, he could feel justified in getting "sexual relief" elsewhere. You don't know what he'll do, but living with ambiguity is part of being a grown-up. Are you going to have sex with him because you're scared he's going to call Betty Sue? Does that make sense? Is that practical? That's the mind-set we've been struggling against since we began the Program, but I wonder how many terms of celibacy have ended because of this fear. Probably too many.

In the final chapter I discuss ending your celibacy intelligently and decisively, but it needs to be stated here and now that ultimately the two of you will have to discuss this important step. Although you are still responsible for your promise to yourself, you are now involved with someone else. You must still be a woman of your word, but you can't just tune him out because you made a promise to yourself. This may be a critical juncture in your relationship: Either you have sex—or not, which may or may not mean the end of the relationship. Only you can decide for yourself what the answer will be.

As you're progressing through your relationship, remembering the following elements will strengthen your chances for success:

+ *Be patient.* Celibacy may be a brave new world for your man, and chances are, you've been at it longer than he has. It may take a while for him to achieve his own comfort level. He may be angry, frustrated, and afraid. As we've seen in this chapter, men are dealing with myriad identity and emotional issues, and celibacy will, no doubt, bring your man face-to-face with them. Reassure him that despite your stand on celibacy, you think that he's the sexiest man on the planet. Let him know how attractive you find him and how flattered you are by his attention.

✦ *Talk, talk, talk.* The more the two of you talk about matters of the heart, mind, and body, the greater your potential for intimacy and lasting happiness.

✦ *Respect his physical boundaries and don't forget your own.* Necking and petting are common among couples practicing celibacy, but don't push him into deeper waters if he tells you that the point of no return—sexual intercourse—is near. Sometimes women can handle deeper hugs and kisses without giving in to the urge to have intercourse, but beware: Men are truly programmed for penile penetration. Use restraint, and he'll follow your lead.

✦ *Discover the vastness of the play spectrum together.* Watch movies together and hold hands. Get up before the crack of dawn and have breakfast together, or watch the sunrise. Men love video games; check out the arcade with him. Fly kites together. Advanced couples can take a trip together (with separate rooms). Go exploring together. Ride bikes together. Play miniature golf or go bowling together. Take long walks together. Go dancing. Have fun!

✦ *Set curfews.* By now, you're probably going over to each other's homes, and even though you're actively practicing celibacy, there is still the risk of accidentally landing in bed. Set a curfew on when it's time to go home. If you let him stay over too late and he gets sleepy, then where's he going to sleep? In your bed? Especially in the early stages, this is much too risky.

✦ *Be honest.* Let's say that your man is pressuring you to have sex. You want it too, but mentally, you're not quite there yet. He stops calling as much, and you sense that his attention is drifting. To try and rein him back in, you tell him that you're ready to make love—but not tonight. He wants to set a date, but for the next few days you put him off. Deep down, you know you're still not ready, but you don't want to lose him either, so you keep lying.

Now we're always accusing men of lying, but how often have we been guilty of the same thing? You owe it to yourself, your man, and the relationship that you are growing together to be honest. For some, this will separate the women from the girls.

✦ *Have the courage of your convictions.* Initially your man may not get the point of celibacy. Learn how to discuss your beliefs in a way that is clear and nonjudgmental. People practicing celibacy often feel morally superior to people who choose to have sexually active lifestyles. Get off your high horse and get real with him. Tell him why you decided to become celibate in the first place.

SHARED LAUGHTER
IS EROTIC, TOO.
—MARGE PIERCY

✦ Give him the benefit of the doubt; hopefully, he will respect you for your decision and your self-improvement efforts.

AFFIRMATION: *Saying no to sex for a while has allowed me to get to know men as human beings. I am grateful for my male friendships.*

CHAPTER ELEVEN

Step 9—
Model a Healthy,
Happy
Celibate Lifestyle

*[Mama] tried to teach us about sexual exploitation, but not
at the expense of our sexuality. Mama actually wanted us to
enjoy sex. But at the right time.*

—Gloria Wade-Gayles, "Sexual Beatitudes" in
Pushed Back to Strength

Whether you decide to keep your new lifestyle a secret or shout it from the rooftops is entirely your decision. Just keep in mind that regardless of how you choose to handle it, people will be watching you—especially as you begin to make improvements in your life. Change always gets people's attention, and when they start asking you questions, how are you going to handle it?

You can always choose to say "none of your business," or smile and act mysterious, but consider talking about celibacy if asked. The more you talk about it to believers and skeptics alike, the more comfortable you'll feel about your convictions.

I have always enjoyed my privacy, believe it or not, so when I first started talking about celibacy, it was difficult. Talk to single women about celibacy, and they'll raise their eyebrows, intrigued. Some women laugh with me (or at me) when I talk about it, while others strongly agree with the practice. Of the women who agree with my stand, there are a few who don't agree with my style of celibacy. I'm not religious enough.

Talk to the average man, and he'll look at you with genuine puzzlement. Men act like they don't know what you're talking about. (Many men don't want to know.) Some men feel threatened by a sensuous, sexy woman who is using her time off from sex to improve herself and heal from past wounds. Others are genuinely intrigued.

I MARRIED THE FIRST MAN I EVER KISSED. WHEN I TELL MY CHILDREN THAT, THEY JUST ABOUT THROW UP.

—BARBARA BUSH

Talk to young people about celibacy, and they're interested, even if they've been sexually active. Deep down, most of them, males and females, know they aren't ready, but they don't know how to deal with the pressure of a love interest or peers.

Talk to people who work with sexually active young people, and you'll hear put-downs of celibacy as well as overly liberal acceptance of sexual activity ("give them free condoms because they're going to have sex anyway").

For a lifestyle that is so hidden in the closet, folks sure do have some strong opinions about celibacy. How we carry ourselves during our term of celibacy is very important. If we go around looking depressed, frustrated, and desperate, either we'll attract like-minded people, or folks will run away.

Steps 1 through 6 of the Sensual Celibacy Program focused on self-development and introspection. Steps 7 through 9 are about your relationships to others who will be affected by your practice of celibacy. In this chapter, we'll explore how your positive approach to sexual abstinence can positively affect others, specifically young people. It is important to talk about youth and sexuality because today there is a rise of pregnancy rates and sexually transmitted diseases among teens. This is the most educated generation regarding sex, but it is also a most troubled one. If you are a mother, a woman who works with young people, or someone who is concerned about the future generation, this chapter will give you strategies for dealing with young people and sex.

Feminists vs. the Fundamentalists

Given our own uncertainty around sexual matters, it is no big mystery to me why pregnancy rates and STDs among young people have skyrocketed in the past few years. If we adults haven't learned how to say no to sex that lacks the proper context, why should we expect our children to be more responsible? Most teens want to abstain, but according to the *Macmillan Visual Almanac,* by the age of eighteen, "at least 73% of American boys and 56% of American girls have had intercourse. Fewer than 20% remain virgins throughout their teenage years." Teens want to say no, but for some strange reason they have not developed the resistance skills or the internal will to say no.

Although I am not a card-carrying member of the feminist movement, I do appreciate and acknowledge these women's courageous fights against unequal pay for equal work, sexual harassment, domestic violence, rape (marital and otherwise), incest, and genital mutilation. What I don't understand is the feminist stand on youth sexuality. Abstinence represents a "choice," a key word in the feminist lexicon. However, in the "Virgins and Sluts" issue of *Ms.* magazine, Erica Werner calls the virginity movement a "cult." In another article by Naomi Wolf entitled "The Making of a Slut," Wolf romanticizes girls who have had premarital sex. Werner's article makes the hundreds of thousands of teens who pledge virginity appear silly and manipulated. Wolf's "sluts" are crafted to elicit our sympathy.

First of all, I don't believe in calling girls "sluts," "hoes," or "bitches." That they are having sex at such an early age and with so many uncaring, uncommitted boys indicates that these girls are in trouble and in need of our help, not our romanticizing.

When help comes along, such as the Christian-led virginity movement, feminists trash it instead of seeing the possibilities for good inherent in it. No, I don't agree with the dogma, but apparently the fundamentalists are doing something right.

Feminists advocate secular education over the church-based approach. But according to teen pregnancy and STD statistics, secular education has proven to be a dismal failure. We adults have access to information and still we continue to make unwise decisions. Right now as you read these words, some woman is rubbing the sleep out of her eyes, wondering how she let sex happen with an uncommitted partner who could care less about her. Why should we expect our children to make reasoned decisions when we have such difficulty? Teaching teens about the mechanics of sex and "safer" sex measures against sexually transmitted diseases and handing out free condoms will not prevent teens from having sex. If you don't believe me, call Planned Parenthood or a social service agency in your community to find out how they're doing in the fight to halt the rise in teen pregnancies and STDs. The problems are getting worse, not better, with the current approach of secular education.

Ms. magazine's polarization of these two seemingly opposite lifestyles—abstinence and sexual activity—does not serve our girls. Childhood experiences of abuse and fear could be underlying both. The fact is, fundamentalists have made some headway into the problem. I applaud them for taking a stand. The teen virginity movement is revolutionary and can stem the tide of broken hearts, unwanted pregnancies, STDs, and messed-up lives.

The fundamentalist approach does have some drawbacks, however. The most publicized strategy to get kids to commit to abstaining from sex has been to get them to sign pledge cards. Signing pledge cards alone won't do it. Fear-based hell and brimstone preaching won't do it. Cutesie slogans such as "pet your dog, not a girl" will probably not hold with our world-weary teens.

The slogan "I miss my virginity" is particularly pernicious. It sets up that elitist hierarchy of girls and women that I hated so much during my church days. The slogan also encourages feelings of low self-worth among girls who have had sex. Girls who have had sex too soon do not need romanticizing or judgment—they need our love, support, and counsel. Girls and boys need resistance strategies they can use and still save face among their peers.

While the fundamentalist fear-based approach may work with some kids, I don't think it will work for most kids. Without daily, consistent follow-up and positive reinforcement from family and members of the community, the effort will fail. Yvonne Butchee runs a weekly rap group for girls in one of Chicago's more notorious HUD projects. She laments the fact that once a week is not enough to reinforce the positive prevention and resistance strategies she tries to teach them. In fact, in her first group of girls, nearly all became pregnant over a three-year period. The one who didn't had a vision of going to college and refused to let anything or anyone get in her way. Yvonne says that her girls, and others like them, need someone to hold their hands every day. In homes where parent(s) work, are substance users, or are otherwise unavailable for their children, the children may have lots of unsupervised time on their hands. It is during these moments that they are most vulnerable to having sex and engaging in other risky behaviors, such as drinking alcohol and doing drugs. Supervision and meaningful activities are needed to keep them out of trouble.

Lest we delude ourselves into thinking that the problems are just with inner-city youth, girls from suburbs, small towns, and rural communities are showing up with the same problems. The problems cross geographic, racial, ethnic, and religious boundaries.

My parents kept me and my sisters so busy that we hardly had time to breathe. There were music and dance lessons and pageant competitions. We participated in many school activities. Both of my parents worked as teachers, so I was fortunate; there was always an adult present when I got home from school.

However, the hell and brimstone preaching did not hold for us, nor many of the other girls of my era. As soon as I left home and abandoned the church the first time, my virginity became a thing of the past. A friend who remained a Ten Commandments Celibate until marriage suffered a crisis in faith during her marriage, and upon her bitter divorce proceeded to embark on a wild and dangerous sexual spree. She left her church and abandoned her support network.

Fundamentalists often rely on fear and shaming tactics. They may work initially, but what if a child leaves the church or separates from his support network? This is a quick-fix approach that becomes less effective over time and can damage the psychological health of boys and girls. When sex is linked to concepts such as "original sin" and feminine submission, so many unhealthy connotations are linked to the sex act itself that its beauty becomes obscured under the weight of religious dogma.

*I*N A SURVEY ENTI-
TLED "HELPING
TEENAGERS POSTPONE
SEXUAL INVOLVE-
MENT," M. HOWARD
AND J. B. MCCABE OF
EMORY UNIVERSITY
FOUND THAT 85 PER-
CENT OF SEXUALLY AC-
TIVE FEMALE TEENS
WANTED TO LEARN HOW
TO SAY NO WITHOUT
HURTING THE OTHER
PERSON'S FEELINGS.

—THE BUCKNELLIAN

In addition, though the virginity movement creates a powerful network (peer group) of teens supporting teens, what happens when a child's network disperses? One-shot conventions and workshops do a good job of creating excitement, but the true test and the real work occur at home, on the streets, at school. If there is no communitywide effort to reinforce the abstinence pledges, there's a good chance that teens will have sex before they're ready.

Rather than throwing out the successes of the fundamentalists, I challenge the feminists, many of whom are mothers, to develop an abstinence program for girls and boys, one that is based on our knowledge of the social, psychological, and sexual developmental stages of children and youth. Let's study the virginity movement to see what they're doing right and build on that. Throw out what we abhor. Werner's assertion that the virginity movement "belongs ideologically with the religious right" is wrong. That's like saying celibacy is for Christians, Jews, Muslims, or Buddhists. They may have claimed it, but it does not belong to them. The choice to practice celibacy or remain virgins until marriage or within the context of a loving, committed, healthy *adult* relationship is available to anyone, whether atheist, fundamentalist Christian, or anywhere along the spectrum.

Nearly all adolescents and teens in U.S. public schools are receiving some form of sex education. They have the information. They know all about HIV and STDs. They know that sex can lead to pregnancy. According to many surveys, they even want to practice abstinence. What our children lack is the experience and maturity to make sound decisions. That's where adults come in, but if we're unsure of our position, how can we ever hope to convince our children of the benefits of waiting?

Why is it that we have high expectations regarding our children's academic performance, but vacillate on the question of too soon sexual involvement? Let's have high standards for both. From 1993 to 1996, I worked for the government-funded Safe and Drug-Free Schools and Communities Program. We believed that *any* alcohol or drug use among youth was abuse. We had a zero-use goal. Never once did we rationalize substance use by saying that children would be children. We did not waste our time in designing strategies that provided for some use among some teens. We set our sights high: No substance use among children. Educators, ministers, parents, students—everyone—agreed with this position.

Yet when it comes to sexual abstinence, we'll say boys will be boys, or we teach youth "safe" sex since "they're going to do it anyway." Parents who wouldn't let their children into the house with grades lower than a C will allow their children to have sexual intercourse. Sometimes in their own house! Some will even give them the condoms and birth control pills! We tell our children that drinking alcohol, smoking cigarettes, and doing drugs will not be tolerated. If we can have such high and unwavering expectations regarding those negative behaviors, then why the vacillation on sex?

I submit that we vacillate on this point because we are unsure of our own position. For years we have said yes to sex even when pregnancy was a risk or we were unsure of the man's love—or even his sexual orientation. But now we do not have only ourselves to think about. Our children are in trouble, and they need our help. The kind of help they need is for you to get your priorities in order. This book was written for you. Nine of the ten steps of the Sensual Celibacy Program were designed for you. Step 9, however, is for our children.

Children are master imitators. If you are a single mother with high expectations for your children, which include sexual abstinence while they are living under your authority, then you must begin to model a healthy, happy practice of celibacy for your children to emulate.

The following are some guidelines for modeling a healthy, happy celibacy practice for your children:

ADDRESS YOUR OWN INNER CONFLICTS. If you don't know where you stand on the sex and youth issue, search your soul. Talk it out with close friends and community members that you admire and respect. Then look at your own sexual behavior and attitudes. Would you want your daughter to have the heartaches that come from casual sex? You can't shelter her from all of life's disappointments, but you can give her a fighting chance by modeling a healthy self-respect for your body and maturity around male-female relationships.

To GET READY FOR WHEN MY DAUGHTER STARTS DATING, I HAVE STARTED A NEIGHBORHOOD WATCH GROUP WITH SOME OF THE OTHER FATHERS WHO ARE SKILLED IN WEAPONRY AND MARTIAL ARTS TO PROTECT THE INTENDED VICTIMS—OUR DAUGHTERS.

—SINBAD

RAISE EXPECTATIONS. As was stated before, we expect our children to be good students and to be on their best behavior when company comes to visit. Yet, because of the "everybody's doing it" attitude about sex, we shrug our shoulders helplessly and pray that they don't get pregnant. Some mothers I know will tell their sons and daughters to "not bring any babies home," but they fail to teach them resistance skills and responsibility for their bodies. Raising expectations without teaching them resistance skills or addressing issues of low self-worth is a setup for failure. Take the time to work with your children. They're worth it.

ESTABLISH HOUSE RULES. If you do not set boundaries for your children, the media, gangs, and peer groups will. Introduce house rules for your children from early childhood. The following rules were written with sexual behavior in mind. However, consider establishing a rules chart for all life areas. Discuss the rules with your children. Tell them that the rules exist not to make their lives miserable, but to help them grow to become happy, healthy, and productive men and women.

Rule 1: As long as your children are living under your roof, they are not allowed to have sex.

Rule 2: Children are not allowed to have members of the opposite sex sleep with them in your house.

Rule 3: Children are not allowed to date until fifteen years of age, and then only on double dates or chaperoned dates.

Rule 4: Children are not allowed to go to unchaperoned parties.

Rule 5: Children must return home from dates by 11 P.M. (Check to make sure your curfew meets curfew laws, if any, in your community.)

LIMIT THE NUMBER OF MEN WHO ARE ALLOWED TO MEET YOUR CHILDREN. Model responsible behavior. Platonic male friends are fine, but I've decided not to let any man that I'm casually dating meet and spend time with my kids until I am pretty sure that the relationship is leading to marriage. Why? When you break up with a man, so do your children. The effect on them can be just as devastating as the effect on you. Says Lynne, whose father had several girlfriends during her childhood, "When my father would break up with a woman, it was like getting a divorce each time."

DON'T ALLOW MEN TO SLEEP OVER AT YOUR HOUSE— NOT EVEN YOUR FIANCÉ. Your children are watching your every move. They will feel there is a double standard if you're telling them to abstain and you're having sex. They will not trust you. You may balk at my suggestions to send your fiancé home, but if your relationship does not work out, your children might get the notion that this was casual sex after all, and if Mom can have casual sex, then so can they. For Ten Commandments Celibates, this guideline should not be difficult. As for Technical and Moderate Celibates who eventually decide to become sexually active, find ways to spend time alone away from the kids. If you can't get away, then don't have sex.

ENCOURAGE AND HELP YOUR TEENS FORM A PEER SUPPORT GROUP. Offer the kids free food and they'll come every week. (Get their parents' permission to participate first.) They'll jump at the chance to talk about sexual issues openly and honestly. Don't judge. Just listen.

TALK OPENLY AND FREELY ABOUT SEX TO YOUR CHILDREN. As girls, many of us learned about sex from peers, health class, or a book our mother gave us. A few of our mothers had an enlightened approach to passing on the womanly wisdom, but most felt uncomfortable talking about it. What saved many teens from having sex was the social stigma. We feared the loss of our reputations as "good girls," and we dreaded pregnancy. We were also saved by the fact that so much of our time outside of school was supervised.

Today, there is no such stigma attached to young people having sex or getting pregnant, and with both parents working, their extracurricular time is largely unsupervised. Moreover, our children are being carelessly exposed to sexual commercials during prime time and stories about presidential semen, oral sex, and adultery on the news. I was in the car with my children listening to the news when all of a sudden, the newscaster started talking about the President having oral sex with an intern. Was it really necessary to keep saying "oral sex"? Wasn't it enough to know that the President had gotten caught in a compromising position and then lied about it? Did we have to know all the sexual details? At the very least, couldn't the sexual details have been reserved for discussion on late night television and radio?

As a result of their hearing that newscast, I had to talk to my children about the political drama in ways that was appropriate to their age levels. My six-year-old and I talked about the importance of telling the truth and being true to your husband or wife. I didn't think that she had caught the "oral sex" reference, but I stayed alert to any confusion or questions on her part. Since I knew that the oral-sex remark had not been lost on my twelve-year-old son, with a deep sigh, I brought it up. I knew we had to talk about it, and we did. Turns out he already knew about it. Had read it in a health book somewhere.

If you are squeamish about talking to your children about sex, get over it! You cannot afford to let anyone else teach them about sex but you. And when you talk to them, make sure you stress the importance of abstinence. Single mothers, tell your children that you are practicing celibacy because you love yourself and that you are holding them to the same standard of behavior.

Ultimately, your children will grow up and make their own decisions, but it is up to you to give them a firm foundation. Let them hear the real deal about sex, love, emotions, relationships, and abstinence from you. Then hear them out. Let them talk. Even if they bring up issues that disturb you, practice your poker face on them. Talk to them straight, because more than likely, they've already heard way more than they should.

IF YOU DON'T HAVE A CHILD, VOLUNTEER TO WORK WITH KIDS. Volunteer as a Big Sister. Stress sexual abstinence. Even if your Little Sister continues to have sex, talk to her about it anyway. This might be the first message on abstinence she's ever received. Host a weekly rap session for girls through your local parks district, community recreation center, or church.

LEARN, THEN TEACH RESISTANCE SKILLS. Part of resisting risky behaviors is knowing what to say when opportunities to experiment with sex, drugs, alcohol, etc., arise. Help your children come up with responses to invitations to participate in problematic behavior. Role-play with them so they will become more comfortable with saying no and so they are firm in their position.

EXPERIENCE TV, COMIC BOOKS, VIDEO GAMES, MOVIES, AND MUSIC WITH YOUR CHILDREN. Parents, do you know what media images and themes your child is being exposed to every day? Every once in a while, don't just tell your teen to turn off that loud music, ask him to explain it to you. Have a discussion about the lyrics. Same thing with TV shows and movies.

DEEPEN YOUR RELATIONSHIP WITH YOUR TEENS. As children get older, parents tend to spend less time with them when really just the opposite is needed. Be kind to them. Laugh with them. Kiss and hug them a lot. Listen to them.

TEACH YOUR CHILDREN HOW TO INFUSE SPIRITUALITY INTO THEIR VIRGINITY/ABSTINENCE. There is a difference between religion and spirituality. Organized religion seeks to systematize the worship of God. Spirituality has nothing to do with dogma or theology and everything to do with the courageous following of the Inner Voice. Teach your children how to draw upon their own inner resources of courage, healing, strength, will, self-love, integrity, and their own sense of the sacred to strengthen their resolve to keep their commitment to abstain. Whether you practice a religion or not, teach your children how to pray and hear Spirit for themselves. Show them how to enjoy being quiet. Expose them early on to a love of nature.

 FAST WORD ABOUT ORAL CONTRA-CEPTION. I ASKED A GIRL TO GO TO BED WITH ME AND SHE SAID NO.

—WOODY ALLEN

REINFORCE/REWARD GOOD BEHAVIOR. When your kids do well, tell them! Celebrate! Many of our parents were overly critical of us when we were growing up. Sometimes we felt like we just couldn't do anything right. This, of course, contributes to feelings of stress, depression, and low self-worth. If your kids communicate with you about sexual issues, thank God they're talking to you and not the boy down the street. Positive reinforcement is important to a child's developing sense of self.

MIND YOUR OWN APPEARANCE. If your children see you looking depressed all the time, if your hair is never combed and you wear clothes that make you look old, tired, and frumpy, they're going to get the message that celibacy is a drag. For your own sake as well as theirs, inventory your closet. Update old looks. Get a youthful-looking haircut. If you're not working out and eating healthily, start today. You should never let the lack of a man in your life give you an excuse to let your appearance go. *You* are reason enough to look gorgeous every day.

AFFIRMATION: *I am strong in my convictions about postponing sex, so I feel good about helping a young person sort through his or her questions. Whether or not I have a child, I can make this contribution. I feel good about it.*

CHAPTER TWELVE

Step 10—
End Intelligently
and Decisively

When the enchanted woman has come into her power, then and only then has she the inner strength to turn her face toward someone else. Only then does she have the authority to meet another person's gaze and hold it.

—Marianne Williams, *A Woman's Worth*

＊　＊　＊

Toward the end of my marriage, my ex-husband told me that I would never find anyone else to love me. A horrible thing to say, but at the time, I just wanted out, so I let his words wash over me—or so I thought. Now I understand that this enraged prophecy, this curse pronounced, would accurately describe the quality of my relationships for years to come. How could he have known about the broken promises and heartaches that would dominate my love life? I know how to practice celibacy, raise children, run a business, and more, but love relationships elude and confound me.

Earlier I said that we women practicing celibacy are often the walking wounded. Out of our element as spouse, lover, and soul mate, living in a society that not only ridicules celibacy but makes no provisions to eliminate the need for it, we women can only throw up our hands at times—despite our Sensual Celibacy skills and lessons learned—and beg for mercy.

Despite the difficulties along the way, the Program has been a blessing for me, and I hope for you too. I hope that by now you understand that even though some areas of your life may be improving, you still may experience loneliness from time to time. The void still exists. We sensual celibates miss the blending of minds, bodies, and souls into one single ecstatic act. Sex within the context of a committed, monogamous, healthy, loving relationship allows us to transcend the body and connect with something holy, cosmic, and heavenly in the beloved and in the universe. Most of all, we miss the companionship, intimacy, and love of a worthy man.

The Sensual Celibacy Program stands alone as one of the few, if not the only, quality programs designed to escort women through this time, but in no way can it substitute for the love of a good man. For those women who have walked the same road, you know this to be true. Not all women practicing celibacy find the transition from being single to being part of a couple difficult, but for those of us who just can't seem to get it right, this final chapter is for you.

If you crave a relationship but have been single and/or celibate for eternity, you're what is known as a *chronically single woman*. Karen Jenkins coined this term in her book *Chronically Single Women: How to Get Out of the Singles Trap*. She defines a chronically single woman as one "who at least thinks she wants to be in a committed, intimate relationship but finds herself persistently or repeatedly alone, or involved in relationships that cannot progress into commitment." Jenkins, herself a recovered chronically single woman (she finally met a good man and got married), discusses the many ways women sabotage their own best efforts at finding and maintaining relationships with good men.

I have talked to celibate women and men who have been not only celibate but celibate and single for *years*. How long is too long? It's been about twelve years since my divorce, and even though I've had involvements with men, none have lasted. That's chronically single. Two years may feel too long. It's an entirely personal matter.

How did years go by with you running in the same spot? Without a healthy celibacy practice, you run the risk of becoming chronically single. Or maybe a celibate lifestyle naturally evolved out of your difficulties in relationships. Either way, your singleness has gone on a little too long and you're really beginning to get worried. You may make a good show for your public, but in the aloneness and loneliness of your bedroom at night, you know the true story.

If you didn't crave companionship with a man, being celibate wouldn't pose such a problem. The reality is, you do. Being single can be a great experience, but when it just drags on and on, it can cause great discomfort and pain.

How do you know if you're chronically single? The following clues are based on my own ongoing unraveling of dating and mating fears. You are chronically single if you believe that . . .

+ Watching TV alone on a Saturday night is more fun than going out and meeting new men friends.

+ No man would ever want you at your weight.

+ Men are like kids in a candy store when it comes to meeting and dating women. So many women, so much time to pick and choose.

+ You must compete against other women to find love and happiness with a man.

+ Men don't like women with children.

+ Men aren't emotionally mature enough to handle a woman with needs.

+ Men are threatened by your intelligence and strength.

+ Men are mean.

+ Men evade, men lie, men cheat.

+ Love is painful.

+ Sex is dangerous.

+ Men are frightened off by women who want monogamy and commitment.

If you've been single for a long time and you agree with three or more of these statements, you are probably a chronically single woman. In fact, you probably have your own negative beliefs that you can add to the list. We pay lip service to wanting love and romance, but the truth is, our beliefs and fears often undermine our best efforts. If you have any of these beliefs, make a commitment to root them out of your soul. Look at them, feel the pain, then let them go. How? Resist the negative thoughts. Every time one tries to come up, replace it with a positive one. Recall an event in which you had a positive experience with a man. Recently, I had a blowout on the expressway, and just as I was starting to feel panicky about having to change my own tire, who walks up but an angel of a man. Not only did he change my tire, but he refused to take any money from me. Every time I'm tempted to feel fear and anger about men, I try and remember him. I think about my father and thank my God for his goodness.

Also, watch your conversation, because your words have power. Refuse to get into negative conversations with women friends. It's one thing to try to analyze a relationship, but it's another to tear men down just for the hell of it. The moment your girlfriend opens her mouth to say, "Men are dogs," tell her, "Don't go there." The immediate gratification of a self-righteous rant is not worth long-term anger, bitterness, and loneliness.

I highly recommend Jenkins's book. The psychological model that she presents allows chronically single women to view their situation as a condition to be healed, not a social or feminine inadequacy (i.e., "She's not 'woman enough' to keep a man"). This is not one of those "how to get a man" books, but "how to be the woman you're destined to be" books. In this new model, women are responsible for their own lives and, thus, their healing. No longer can women point to statistics that "prove" the lack of eligible men, nor can they solely blame the men in their lives for their distress. The model Jenkins describes shines the spotlight directly on women's behaviors and subconscious motivations.

Counseling is necessary to break out of the singles rut. A rut is caused by going over the same ground again and again. Sometimes all that's needed is a good push to get you unstuck. The singles rut is prolonged when we refuse, for whatever reasons, to seek help. Alone, you may not be able to clearly see the forces that have created the wall between you and the man of your dreams. Clearly, the fact that you are still alone after so many years and relationships (or maybe no relationships) means that in some fundamental way, your singleness has served you—despite your conscious desire for love and companionship. Ask a qualified therapist to help you figure it out.

Jenkins identifies fear, shame, and inhibition as the great enemies of lasting love. Fear has paralyzed many a chronically single woman, and that fear manifests itself in many ways. Some chronically single women constantly find themselves in and out of relationships. They never stay long enough to let themselves be known. Others—and I believe this is where many celibate women come in—rarely make a move outside their homes except to go to work and the grocery store. Their sedentary lifestyles lead to obesity and related chronic ailments. Many fill their lives with busywork that has nothing to do with life mission and everything to do with hiding from the root causes of their souls' ache. A chronically single woman may have an affair with a married or otherwise unavailable man. Or she may keep a "maintenance man" until Mr. Right comes along. The common denominator connecting all these women is their fear, shame, and inhibition that prevent them from finding and maintaining that one quality relationship they so desperately desire.

If you suspect that you are using celibacy as a way to escape from life and from interaction with others, you might be a chronically single woman. You may think you're coping—maybe you are, but you're not living. A qualified counselor will help you unravel the root causes of your fears. She will also help you correct self-defeating behaviors. Seeking help is a supreme act of self-love and a critical step to addressing your soul's need for a lasting love relationship.

Most important, you must know without a doubt that you are "woman enough" to love a man and maintain a healthy, monogamous, committed love relationship. That you have not says nothing about your value as a woman. Look at everything else you're doing: maintaining a household, socializing, improving your mind and body, working, volunteering, running a business or developing your career, or single parenting. It's only this one area that's got you stumped. That's no crime. The people (usually women) who judge you and say you're not woman enough, what have they done with their lives? Okay, so they can get on the Ricki Lake show and say, "I got a man." So what! *I got a life.* A man will come at the right time.

LIVING TO A RIPE OLD AGE IS EASY—JUST CUT OUT FOOD AND SEX!

—HEADLINE FROM THE *NATIONAL ENQUIRER*, OCTOBER 8, 1996

"YOU'RE TALKING ABOUT A LIFE SPAN OF ALMOST 170," GEORGE ROTH, A SCIENTIST AT THE NATIONAL INSTITUTE ON AGING IS QUOTED AS SAYING.

In step one, you began your celibacy practice with a decision. In this final step of the Sensual Celibacy Program, you end the same way: with a decision.

Let's say that your relationship is getting serious. For Ten Commandments Celibates who are firm in their resolve, the answer is easy: No sex until marriage. But for Moderate and Technical Celibates, the decision to end a term of celibacy may not be as clear-cut. Normally, a woman lets her sexual urges and/or external pressure ("please, baby, please") lead her into a sexual rendezvous, but desire is not enough. You may feel that being rational and logical about something as wild and woolly as sex will take away from the excitement. Better to step back and reflect a moment than to make a decision you'll regret. If your most pressing questions about the course and future of your relationship haven't yet been answered, don't have sex hoping that the physical intimacy will eventually smooth and sort everything out. It won't. In addition to answering the questions that are unique to your relationship, you'll need to know the following:

+ What kind of birth control will you both be using? Has he agreed to use a condom?

+ If he does not want to use a condom, can he produce the results of an HIV test? Can he prove that he doesn't have herpes or any other STDs?

+ If you do get pregnant, what will you do? If you choose to keep the baby, what will be his role in the child's life—father/husband or child supporter/baby-sitter?

+ What are his long-term intentions toward you? If he does not see marriage in his future, will you still agree to have sex? If he says he does want marriage, just not right now, then when? And does that mean he wants to marry *you*? Has he bought you a ring?

+ How much has he involved you in his life? Have you met his family? Has he introduced you to coworkers and friends?

Good decision making requires intelligence, common sense, and information. If only women had access to better information about the men who cross their paths, we'd make better decisions. Unfortunately, very few men will admit to only wanting a good jack. Typically, there'll be a lot of dancing and romancing and outright avoidance of the topic. The only way you're going to get the information you need is to talk to your man. Ask him questions. Without a doubt, I've been plenty afraid of appearing too nosey, but how else are you going to find out what you need to know unless you ask questions? As he talks, be quiet and *listen* to what he says and then watch what he does. If answers are not forthcoming, or if his behavior conflicts with his words, then don't end your celibacy practice just yet. If, on the other hand, you like what you hear and see, then you've got a winner.

Trust your instincts. If despite your love and sexual desire for a man you can't shake the feeling that something is not quite right, don't ignore the feeling. Pay attention to what your gut is telling you. This may sound obvious, but how often have we ignored the warnings of the still small Voice for a moment of pleasure that turned out disastrous? Stay awake. Don't go on automatic.

Years ago I knew a young woman who decided that she was tired of being a virgin. She had been in a relationship with a man that she liked a lot, and chose him to help her make the transition into sexual womanhood. What I loved about her handling of this most delicate affair was that she never once went on automatic and accidentally had sex in the back of that man's car. She made a decision then ritualized it by planning contraception, telling her friends about what she intended to do, and buying sexy lingerie for the occasion.

You may be ready to end your term of celibacy even though there's no man in sight. That's okay too. For you, the decision to end is a mindset and an act of faith that says you're ready for a healthy, loving, committed, monogamous relationship that includes sex. Whether you're in a relationship or not, the first step to ending your celibacy practice is making the decision.

Next, call up all the members of your support group, and call the individual who signed your Celibacy Promise as a witness. Let them all

I, _____, do on this date of _____
_____ nullify my promise to practice celibacy. By making this decision I am in effect declaring that I'm not only ready for a love relationship, but that I'm ready to have sex.

_____
Signed   Date

_____
Witness (optional)   Date

know that you've decided to end your term of celibacy. They will probably have a long list of questions for you. Don't hang up on them. They're only doing their job. Listen to them carefully: They may come up with angles that you hadn't considered.

Then announce your intention to the Universe:

Thank you for sending me my soul mate. I ask for your blessing as I enter into this sexual dimension of our relationship. Let our love grow like the flowers in your holy garden, and let sex only serve to deepen the incredible intimacy we already share. I thank you for the experience and blessing of my celibacy practice. As I leave it today, I will never forget to carry with me forever and ever the lessons I learned and the healing that I gained. I thank you for the wonderful blessings of love, monogamy, commitment, and marriage. Let your love flood us and make us one healthy interdependent couple. Thank you. And So It Is.

If you're ending your term of celibacy as a mind-set, say these words:

Thank you for this gift of celibacy. The time alone healed old wounds and put me on a path that is filled with purpose and meaning. As an act of faith, I now end this term of celibacy. I am now open and willing to receive a love relationship that brings sex into my life. In the name of all that is holy, I intend for this to be a monogamous, healthy, committed soul mate relationship that is filled with your love. I thank you. And So It Is.

Now, celebrate with the members of your support group. Throw a party or cook dinner for them. Perform a ritual by yourself that helps you to firmly end your term of celibacy. Perform an act that would signify to you the end of this era. Go to the ocean and throw flowers in the water. Take the Celibacy Promise that you signed at the beginning of this book and burn it with your blessings.

Finally, perform a ritual with your man. It could be something as simple and fun as popping red cherries (symbolic of your you-know-what) into each other's mouths. Performing a ritual together will deepen the intimacy between you and reinforce in his mind what a "pearl of great price" he is gaining. He should feel more loving and protective of you. You should feel cherished and beautiful.

Congratulations! May your transition into your new life be filled with satisfaction, beauty, and love.

I believe with all my heart that if you work it, the Sensual Celibacy Program will help you get your life in order and deepen your intimacy with men. Its emphasis on self-knowledge aims to get to the root of and address our souls' discontent. Its emphasis on gratitude, forgiveness, inner healing, mission, and self-love has the power to change us from the inside out. That's not to say that a similar process cannot occur in the context of relationship: It can, and many fine doctors of the soul are passionately working in that arena to help couples work out their problems.

For the millions of women and men (one-third of the adult population, as Shere Hite says) not in a relationship and not having sex, the opportunity is a golden one to address the needs of the soul, to retrieve fragments of the soul that were lost or stolen in childhood, to burn the tapes of obsolete subconscious programming.

The Sensual Celibacy Program may not be for all single people—not even all practicing celibates. Still, I hope that you will take with you a message of hope. I wrote Sensual Celibacy because every adult woman and man I have ever known has experienced at least one heartbreak in a love relationship. As wonderful as it is, sex is the powder keg that can blow up in a couple's face—if the development of friendship and intimacy does not occur first. This book is my own personal white flag of surrender. I no longer care to be right; I just want love, peace, and harmony to reign among us. Male and female bashing serves no one. I have participated in those conversations that rake men over the coals, but it does not heal my soul to put men down. All it does is stir up the anger. I'm tired of being pissed off. I want to make love, not war.

So as I date and risk rejection and learn to love again, I am in awe of the resiliency of the human spirit. I've suffered so much pain in relationships, but still I hope and pray and wait for my soul mate to hurry up and find me now. I look through the crowds waiting to find that one pair of warm, loving eyes to connect to mine, to hear that one baritone voice whisper in my ear, "Oh, baby."

We celibate women are reluctant, passionate, complex, and wonderful creatures. We are loving. We are lovable. We are love.

The adventure continues.